HEALTH POLICY
AND ECONOMICS:
OPPORTUNITIES
AND CHALLENGES

STATE OF HEALTH SERIES

Edited by Chris Ham, Professor of Health Policy and Management
at the University of Birmingham.

HEALTH POLICY AND ECONOMICS: OPPORTUNITIES AND CHALLENGES

Edited by
**Peter C. Smith,
Laura Ginnelly and
Mark Sculpher**

Open University Press

Open University Press
McGraw-Hill Education
McGraw-Hill House
Shoppenhangers Road
Maidenhead
Berkshire
England
SL6 2QL

email: enquiries@openup.co.uk
world wide web: www.openup.co.uk

and Two Penn Plaza, New York, NY 10121-2289, USA

First published 2005
Reprinted 2011

A catalogue record of this book is available from the British Library

ISBN 0 335 21574 2 (pb) 0 335 21575 0 (hb)

Library of Congress Cataloging-in-Publication Data
CIP data applied for

Typeset by RefineCatch Limited, Bungay, Suffolk
Printed and bound by CPI Group (UK) Ltd, Croydon, CR0 4YY

CONTENTS

LIST OF CONTRIBUTORS

Ron Akehurst is Dean and Professor of Health Economics in the School for Health and Related Research, University of Sheffield.

Karen Bloor is Senior Research Fellow in the Department of Health Sciences, University of York.

Martin Buxton is Professor of Health Economics and Director of the Health Economics Research Group at Brunel University.

Karl Claxton is Senior Lecturer in the Department of Economics and Related Studies and Centre for Health Economics (CHE), University of York.

Richard Cookson is Senior Lecturer in Health Economics in the School of Medicine Health Policy and Practice at the University of East Anglia.

Diane Dawson is Senior Research Fellow in the Centre for Health Economics (CHE), University of York.

Paul Dolan is Professor of Economics at the University of Sheffield.

Mike Drummond is Professor of Health Economics and Director of the Centre for Health Economics (CHE), University of York.

Brian Ferguson is Professor of Health Economics and Director of the Yorkshire & Humber Public Health Observatory, University of York.

Laura Ginnelly is a Research Fellow in the Centre for Health Economics (CHE), University of York.

Maria Goddard is Assistant Director and leads the Health Policy research team at the Centre for Health Economics (CHE), University of York.

Hugh Gravelle is Professor of Economics and leads the National Primary Care Research and Development Centre at the Centre for Health Economics (CHE), University of York.

Katharina Hauck is a Research Fellow in the Centre for Health Economics (CHE), University of York.

John Hutton is Senior Research Leader at MEDTAP International Inc, London.

Rowena Jacobs is a Research Fellow in the Centre for Health Economics (CHE), University of York.

Andrew Jones is Professor of Economics and Director of the Graduate Programme in Health Economics at the Department of Economics and Related Studies, University of York.

Paul Kind is Senior Research Fellow and leads the Outcomes Research Group at the Centre for Health Economics (CHE), University of York.

Rosella Levaggi is Professor of Public Economics in the Department of Economic Sciences at the University of Brescia.

Guillem López Casasnovas is Professor of Economics and Director of the Centre for Research on Economics and Health (CRES) at Pompeu Fabra University.

Alan Maynard is Professor of Health Economics, Department of Health Sciences and Director of the York Health Policy Group, University of York. He is also Chairman of the York NHS Trust.

Nigel Rice is a Reader in Health Economics at the Centre for Health Economics (CHE), University of York.

Anthony Scott is a Reader in Health Economics and Director of the Behaviour, Performance and the Organization of Care Programme at the Health Economics Research Unit, University of Aberdeen.

Mark Sculpher is Professor of Health Economics and leads the team for Economic Evaluation and Health Technology Assessment at the Centre for Health Economics (CHE), University of York.

Rebecca Shaw is a Research Graduate in the Department of Sociology, University of York.

Trevor Sheldon is Professor in the Department of Health Sciences, University of York.

Peter C. Smith is Professor of Economics at the University of York, where he is based in the Centre for Health Economics and the Department of Economics and Related Studies.

Andrew Street is Senior Research Fellow and Assistant Director of the Health Policy Team at the Centre for Health Economics (CHE), University of York.

Matt Sutton is Senior Research Fellow in the Department of General Practice and Primary Care at the University of Glasgow.

Adrian Towse is Director of the Office of Health Economics.

Aki Tsuchiya is Lecturer in Health Economics at the University of Sheffield.

Alan Williams is Professor of Economics at the Centre for Health Economics (CHE), University of York.

SERIES EDITOR'S INTRODUCTION

Health services in many developed countries have come under critical scrutiny in recent years. In part this is because of increasing expenditure, much of it funded from public sources, and the pressure this has put on governments seeking to control public spending. Also important has been the perception that resources allocated to health services are not always deployed in an optimal fashion. Thus at a time when the scope for increasing expenditure is extremely limited, there is a need to search for ways of using existing budgets more efficiently. A further concern has been the desire to ensure access to health care of various groups on an equitable basis. In some countries this has been linked to a wish to enhance patient choice and to make service providers more responsive to patients as 'consumers'.

Underlying these specific concerns are a number of more fundamental developments which have a significant bearing on the performance of health services. Three are worth highlighting. First, there are demographic changes, including the ageing population and the decline in the proportion of the population of working age. These changes will both increase the demand for health care and at the same time limit the ability of health services to respond to this demand.

Second, advances in medical science will also give rise to new demands within the health services. These advances cover a range of possibilities, including innovations in surgery, drug therapy, screening and diagnosis. The pace of innovation quickened as the end of the twentieth century approached, with significant implications for the funding and provision of services.

Third, public expectations of health services are rising as those who use services demand higher standards of care. In part, this is stimulated by developments within the health service, including the availability of new technology. More fundamentally, it stems from the emergence of a more educated and informed population, in which people are accustomed to being treated as consumers rather than patients.

Against this background, policy makers in a number of countries are reviewing the future of health services. Those countries which have traditionally relied on a market in health care are making greater use of regulation and planning. Equally, those countries which have traditionally relied on regulation and planning are moving towards a more competitive approach. In no country is there complete satisfaction with existing methods of financing and delivery, and everywhere there is a search for new policy instruments.

The aim of this series is to contribute to debate about the future of health services through an analysis of major issues in health policy. These issues have been chosen because they are both of current interest and of enduring importance. The series is intended to be accessible to students and informed lay readers as well as to specialists working in this field. The aim is to go beyond a textbook approach to health policy analysis and to encourage authors to move debate about their issues forward. In this sense, each book presents a summary of current research and thinking, and an exploration of future policy directions.

Professor Chris Ham
Professor of Health Policy and Management
University of Birmingham

ACKNOWLEDGEMENTS

Numerous people contributed wittingly or otherwise to the preparation of the book. We must acknowledge the constructive comments of the discussants, some of whom have contributed short commentaries to the book chapters. The participants at the CHE conference provided invaluable observations on many of the contributions. Rachel Gear and Hannah Cooper at Open University Press offered timely support throughout the project. Mike Drummond, the director of CHE, has provided unstinting support throughout, and our colleagues Stephanie Cooper, Helen Parkinson and Trish Smith contributed excellent secretarial and administrative assistance. The contributions of these and others undoubtedly improved considerably the contents of the book, and our thanks are due to all.

INTRODUCTION
Peter C. Smith, Mark Sculpher and Laura Ginnelly

Health policy poses some of the greatest challenges for modern economies. The proportion of gross domestic product (GDP) attributed to health care is growing rapidly in almost all developed countries, yet traditional methods of financing health care are coming under strain. Life expectancies are increasing, but health disparities are an enduring policy issue in many countries. The providers of health care – especially doctors – are uniquely powerful interest groups that policymakers challenge at their peril. New technologies arrive at an accelerating pace, and there are often formidable pressures to adopt them quickly. And the expectations of an increasingly assertive citizenry grow steadily.

These challenges reflect an increasing need to deploy scarce resources to the best possible effect. Management of scarcity is a central preoccupation of the economics discipline, so it is not surprising to find that policymakers have turned to economists for advice. This book documents many of the successful influences of economic ideas on health policy. However, its more important purpose is to look forward to future policy challenges, and to assess the potential contribution economic analysis might make to addressing them. In doing so, we recognize that, when used as a basis for policy analysis in the health field, traditional economic methods often need to be complemented by insights from other perspectives. Where possible, we therefore seek to emphasize the important links with other disciplines.

Modern economics is usually traced back to 1776, when Adam Smith published *The Wealth of Nations*. That work irrevocably associated the discipline with the functioning of markets. However, in the intervening period, economists have sought to extend their purview to almost all aspects of human endeavour. They came to health quite late. The genesis of what we now know as health economics is often said to be the seminal 1963 article by Kenneth Arrow, which sought to apply traditional economic principles to the analysis of health care (Arrow 1963).

Since the publication of Arrow's paper, it has become clear that health and health care offer an abundance of problems to which the tools of economic analysis can be applied, and that the analytic and empirical findings have very important messages for policy. The *Handbook of Health Economics* documents just how extensive the scope and policy impact of economic analysis in the health domain has become (Culyer and Newhouse 2000). The contributions embrace micro models of the behaviour of individual patients and health professionals, evaluative studies of health care organizations, public health and medical interventions, design of financing and incentive mechanisms, and macro issues of law and regulation. A particularly noteworthy characteristic of health economists has been their willingness to work with other disciplines (such as physicians, epidemiologists and statisticians).

In the UK, our colleague Alan Williams was one of the first to realize the potential of economic analysis applied to health, and in a distinguished career has made numerous influential contributions to academic and policy debates (Culyer and Maynard 1997). The Health Economics Study Group met for the first time in York in 1972, as a conscious attempt to establish health economics as a distinct discipline, and has since gone from strength to strength (Croxson 1998). A distinctive feature of the group has been a strong interest in and influence on policy (Hurst 1998). Many nations have established their own health economics associations, and in 1993 the International Health Economics Association was established. It now has about 2500 members and has held four conferences, the third of which was in York in 2002, attracting over 1300 delegates and presentations from two Nobel laureates.

In 1983 the University of York established the Centre for Health Economics (CHE), one of the first research institutes specializing in the economics of health, with Alan Maynard as the first director.[1] The Centre has flourished, and is now led by Mike Drummond. This book arises from a conference held to celebrate the twentieth anniversary of its foundation. At least one author of each conference chapter was a current member of CHE, and each chapter was discussed by a distinguished alumnus or former associate of CHE. We include most of those discussions as postscripts to

the relevant chapter. For obvious reasons, the book focuses especially on UK health policy. However, we have sought to draw out
the implications of our findings for mature health systems of all
sorts.

The logic of the book is to start with micro, patient-level issues
and to progress to macro, whole-system issues. In the concluding
chapter we argue that – at least in principle – the micro/macro
distinction is artificial. However, we hope the reader finds the
progression to be a useful organizing principle. Chapters 1 and 2
therefore address the problem of determining the most cost-effective
forms of management to offer patients. Chapters 3 and 4 then
consider issues of fairness and the distribution of health within the
population. In Chapters 5, 6, 7 and 8, we move on to examine
performance measurement and incentives for organizations and
individual workers. In conclusion, Chapters 9 and 10 examine the
implications of the simultaneous pressures for both increased
decentralization and increased internationalization of health
systems. We conclude this introduction by briefly summarizing the
contribution of each chapter.

Almost all health systems have – either explicitly or implicitly – to
make decisions about which health care programmes and interventions to fund from collective resources. These 'reimbursement
decisions' are in practice unavoidable, even in situations of severe
limitations in the evidence base. In this domain, seeking to select
the most cost-effective interventions has been widely accepted as a
guiding principle. England and Wales has therefore established
the National Institute for Clinical Excellence (NICE) to make such
principles operational, and equivalent institutions are being created
in many other countries.

However, as Sculpher, Claxton and Akehurst (Chapter 1) explain,
the work of such organizations has exposed thorny methodological
issues that have previously not been dealt with explicitly. They argue
that conventional neoclassical welfare economics has limitations in
assessing the value of health care programmes. Rather, the problem
of identifying efficient health care interventions should be seen as
one of constrained maximization. This requires careful definition of
the objective function and of the range of constraints facing the
system. This process, as well as that of synthesizing available
evidence and the analytical tasks of identifying cost-effective
interventions and assessing the value and optimal design of
future research, emphasizes the multi-disciplinary nature of health
technology assessment and economic evaluation.

The valuation of health outcomes is central to the delivery and evaluation of health care. In its infancy, health economics (and its practitioners) demanded intellectually rigorous but simple tools with which to prosecute its science. This resulted in the development of instruments such as quality-adjusted life years (QALYs). The widespread practical acceptance of such methods is, in many respects, a triumph for those researchers. It is also a beacon for other, more mature areas of economic inquiry to emulate. However, as Kind documents (Chapter 2), there remain some important methodological and practical challenges to resolve if the QALY approach is to continue to answer the needs of policymakers in the future.

Disparities in health status and access to health care are dominant themes in many policy debates. However, debates on the concept of fairness are often confused and lacking in rigour, and equity has hitherto played hardly any explicit role in the conduct of economic evaluations of health care technologies. Yet NICE and similar bodies are explicitly charged with taking equity into account. Williams, Tsuchiya and Dolan (Chapter 3) consider how the views of citizens might be elicited in an intellectually coherent manner, such as to be usable by bodies like NICE. The intention is to offer an economic framework within which considerations of efficiency and equity can be balanced.

There is a rich tradition of economic analysis of income inequality. Within this tradition, Jones and Rice (Chapter 4) examine the extent to which health and health care utilization are unequally distributed by income. They argue that only by developing a proper understanding of the causal mechanisms generating these inequalities will it be possible to develop effective policies. Their methods involve the analysis of panel data (repeated observations for individual respondents) rather than the more usual cross-sectional (one-off) survey data. Such data resources are becoming increasingly common, and offer the prospect of gaining important insights into the dynamics of health and its relation to socioeconomic characteristics. The analysis entails the use of advanced econometric techniques which – while challenging in detail to the lay reader – offer the prospect of major advances in policy understanding of inequalities.

Mainstream economics offers numerous prescriptions for the organization and regulation of complex industries. It is therefore somewhat surprising that – outside of the USA – the economics of industrial organization has had little impact on health policy. Cookson, Goddard and Gravelle (Chapter 5) examine the relevance of economic analysis in this domain, and raise questions that policymakers should be asking. Examples of policy issues include the link between the size of organizations and performance, the impact of different risk-sharing arrangements, the design of incentives, the role of private sector providers, the design of purchaser-provider contracts and the implications of patient choice. The chapter demonstrates the importance of having good economic models with which to address such questions and to guide empirical research.

A particularly central concern for empirical work is the need to develop good measures of organizational performance. The *World Health Report 2000*, and subsequent work at the Organization for Economic Co-operation and Development (OECD), has identified performance measurement as a crucial instrument for securing system improvements. Yet health care is in many respects a uniquely complex industry, and many existing measurement instruments are very weak, particularly in the domain of clinical quality. Jacobs and Street (Chapter 6) examine future prospects for the measurement and reporting of organizational performance in health and health care, with a particular emphasis on efficiency measurement. Increasingly, sophisticated econometric tools are being used to draw inferences about organizational efficiency, but are they ready for such use?

Health care is a labour intensive undertaking, so it is hardly surprising that workforce planning and the health labour markets are key concerns for most health systems. The policy concern is heightened by acute labour shortages in some countries. Mainstream economics offers insights into how substitution possibilities and incentives can be used to promote labour force flexibility, encouraging efficient changes in the mix of inputs into the production process. Bloor and Maynard (Chapter 7) demonstrate the importance of rigorous designs in evaluating these issues, illustrated with recent trends and reforms in the UK labour market.

Fair financing is a core issue in all types of health system. Traditionally, the intention has been merely to create a level playing field, with the aim of ensuring that all citizens can gain access to the current standard level of health care (securing horizontal equity). The question of whether the current standard is in line with policy intentions is rarely addressed. However, recent policy in England has shifted to a more radical concept of fair financing, in the form of reducing avoidable health disparities (moving towards vertical equity). Hauck, Shaw and Smith (Chapter 8) examine from a theoretical perspective the implications of this radical change, and highlight the need to introduce explicit incentives to address the causes of premature mortality (or disability) if such finance reforms are to be successful.

Decentralization is an emerging policy theme in many health systems. While countries such as Italy, Spain and the UK are seeking to devolve financing and policy authority to more local institutions, others such as Norway, Poland and Portugal are seeking to centralize powers. The implication of decentralization for the equity and efficiency of public services is one of the central interests of modern public finance theory. It is therefore somewhat surprising that much health policy is formulated without reference to this theory and the associated empirical evidence. Levaggi and Smith (Chapter 9) examine the relevance of mainstream public economics for countries grappling with the problem of seeking to establish the most appropriate level at which to set policy and how best to finance their health system. Rather than offer definitive policy guidance, the contribution of economic theory is to offer a framework within which policymakers can debate decentralization options.

Alongside increased decentralization of national health systems, there is a parallel move towards integration at the supra-national level, most notably in the European Union (EU). Increased integration offers immense challenges for policymakers in the domains of harmonization, regulation and market structure. Dawson, Drummond and Towse (Chapter 10) examine from an economic perspective a number of important developments in European policy. They cite examples such as the move from harmonization of drug licensing towards harmonization of procedures for assessing the cost-effectiveness of health technologies, as well as the increased freedom offered to patients to seek cross-border health care, and trace the associated lessons for policymakers.

In Chapter 11 we draw out a few dominant themes that emerge from the contributions. They include: the pervasive concern with equity, and its link with efficiency; the need for economists to engage with other disciplines if they are to answer policy questions persuasively; and the need to recognize the interconnectedness of the policy questions we have discussed. Major advances have been made in using economic thinking to inform policy, but there remain many challenges. We hope that the book offers some pointers for how those challenges might be addressed.

NOTES

1 The distinction of being the first dedicated health economics research unit (at least in Europe) is claimed by Aberdeen University, which established its Health Economics Research Unit (HERU) in 1977 (Scott *et al.* 2003).

REFERENCES

Arrow, K. (1963) Uncertainty and the welfare economics of medical care, *American Economic Review*, 53(5): 941–73.

Croxson, B. (1998) From private club to professional network: an economic history of the Health Economists' Study Group, 1972–1997, *Health Economics*, 7(suppl): S9–S45.

Culyer, A.J. and Maynard, A.K. (1997) *Being Reasonable about the Economics of Health: Selected Essays by Alan Williams*. Cheltenham: Edward Elgar.

Culyer, A.J. and Newhouse, J.P. (2000) *Handbook of Health Economics*. Amsterdam: Elsevier.

Hurst, J. (1998) The impact of health economics on health, policy in England, and the impact of health policy on health economics, 1972–1997, *Health Economics*, 7(suppl): S47–S61.

Scott, A., Maynard, A. and Elliot, R. (2003) *Advances in Health Economics*. Chichester: Wiley.

1

IT'S JUST EVALUATION FOR DECISION-MAKING: RECENT DEVELOPMENTS IN, AND CHALLENGES FOR, COST-EFFECTIVENESS RESEARCH

Mark Sculpher, Karl Claxton and Ron Akehurst

INTRODUCTION

The history of economic evaluation in health care has been characterized by doubts regarding whether this form of research has any impact on health service decision-making (Duthie *et al.* 1999). Although many questions remain about whether formal analysis is used to inform resource allocation at the level of the individual hospital or practice, economic evaluation is now increasingly used as an input into decisions regarding which interventions and programmes represent good value at the level of the health care system (Hjelmgren *et al.* 2001). In the UK, the explicit use of economic evaluation to inform decision-making has manifested itself most clearly in the National Institute for Clinical Excellence (NICE 2001).

The increasing use of economic evaluation for this purpose partly reflects developments in methods and an increase in rigour in this area of research. Over the last ten years, the methods used in economic evaluation have rapidly developed in areas such as characterizing and handling uncertainty, statistical analysis of patient-level data and the use of decision analysis. There remain, however, significant challenges in the field, and it is essential that the increasing application of economic evaluation to inform decision-making is accompanied by programmes of research on methodology.

This chapter takes a broad view of the 'state of the art' in economic evaluation in health care. It considers three questions: What is the appropriate theoretical foundation and correct analytical framework for economic evaluation, used to inform defined decision problems in health care? Given an appropriate foundation and framework, what are the recent methodological achievements in economic evaluation? What methodological challenges remain to be tacked in the field? To address these questions, the chapter is structured as follows. First, we consider the alternative theoretical foundation for economic evaluation, and argue that a societal decision-making perspective is the most appropriate. We also discuss the requirements for economic evaluation that follow from a focus on societal decision-making. Second, we describe recent methods advances in economic evaluation relating to the generation of evidence: the methods of evidence synthesis, handling uncertainty and prioritizing future research. Third, we consider methods challenges which need to be addressed for economic evaluation to reach its potential. This section focuses on the need to develop a fuller set of analytical tools around constrained maximization and to address key research questions associated with prioritizing and designing future research. Our final section offers some conclusions.

ECONOMIC EVALUATION FOR DECISION-MAKING

The theoretical foundation for economic evaluation

In order to identify the important methods developments in economic evaluation, it is necessary to ascertain what questions these studies should be addressing by identifying an appropriate normative framework for economic evaluation. The strong normative foundation provided by neoclassical welfare economic theory gives clear guidance on what is meant by efficiency, how costs and benefits should be measured, what perspective should be taken and whether a change (adoption of a new health technology) improves social welfare. However, these strong normative prescriptions come at a price in two important ways. First, the values implicit in this framework may not necessarily be shared by a legitimate societal decision-maker or analyst, and are certainly not universally accepted. Second, its application to a presumed nirvana of a first-best neoclassical world, where market prices represent the social value of alternative activities (and, when they do not, they can be shadow-priced assuming a first-best world), only fits with a narrow and rarified view of the world.

As a theoretical framework to guide economic evaluation in health care, welfare economic theory would have a series of implications. The first is that health care programmes should be judged in the same way as any other proposed change. That is, the only question is whether they represent a potential Pareto improvement (as measured by a compensation test), not whether they improve health outcomes as measured, for example, on the basis of health-related quality of life (HRQL). Second, there is an implicit view that the current distribution of income, if not optimal, is at least acceptable (Pauly 1995), and that the distributive impacts of health care programmes, and the failure actually to pay compensation, are negligible. An implicit justification for this view is that the current distribution of income results from individual choices about the trade-offs between work and leisure time and about investing in human capital (Grossman 1972).

In addition, there are a number of substantial problems in the application of the prescriptions of welfare theory: the conditions of rationality and consistency required for individuals maximizing their utility have been shown to be violated in most choice situations (Machina 1987): the problem of aggregating individual compensating variations (Boadway 1974); the paradox of choice reversal with non-marginal changes (Arrow and Scitovsky 1969); issues of path dependency (Green 1976); and the problem of second best (Ng 1983). The last of these has received very little attention, despite the well known, but devastating, result that first-best solutions (and the shadow pricing associated with them) in a second-best world may move us away from a Pareto optimum and not towards one. Since no one would argue that the world is first best, then, even if the values implicit in welfare economic theory were acceptable, its successful application in a second-best world seems implausible.

There is a strong argument, then, that the application of welfare theory to economic evaluation in health care is either impossible or inappropriate or both. The societal decision-making view, in contrast, does not require such a rarified view of the world, is directly relevant, from a societal perspective, to the type of decision-making which economic evaluation is increasingly being asked to inform, and attempts to make explicit the legitimacy of any normative prescriptions based on it.

Of course, it is possible to justify cost-effectiveness analysis (CEA) within a welfare theoretic framework (Garber and Phelps 1997; Meltzer 1997; Weinstein and Manning 1997). However, generally, but particularly in the UK, it is the 'Extra Welfarist' (Culyer 1989), and particularly the societal decision-making, view (Sugden and Williams 1979) which departs from strict adherence to welfare theory, that have implicitly or explicitly provided the methodological foundations of CEA in health. In essence, this approach takes an exogenously defined societal objective and an exogenous budget constraint for health care, and views CEA as providing the technical tools to solve this constrained optimization problem.

It is true, however, that, as currently used, the characterization of the exogenous objective function has been somewhat naïve and limited to maximizing health outcome, often measured by quality-adjusted life years (QALYs). Similarly, the characterization of constraints has been limited to a single budget constraint. If we are to see CEA as a constrained maximization problem from the perspective of a societal decision-maker, then a much more sophisticated characterization of the optimization problem will be required. Also, the required specification of an objective, and the means of measuring, valuing and aggregating health outcomes are not universally accepted. Consequently, unlike welfare theory, the societal decision-making approach to CEA cannot, by itself, provide a strong normative prescription for social choice.

Thus, neither the neoclassical nor the societal decision-making approach can, in practice, provide the all embracing normative framework for CEA that would be desirable. It may be argued, however, that by rooting discussion around the practicalities of decision-making and acknowledging the complexity of the world in which we live, a societal decision-making approach offers the better chance for progress in our understanding of the implications of our choices.

Societal decision-making is certainly the context in which economic evaluation is being increasingly used to inform policy. To be useful, however, CEA must have some normative content. The legitimacy and, therefore, the normative prescriptions of this approach to CEA rest with the legitimacy of the specification of the objective function and the characterization of the constraints. In other words, the solution to this constrained optimization problem requires an external legitimacy to have normative content.

The societal decision-making approach does not imply that CEA should be conducted from the perspective of particular decision-makers, it is possible to have a broad societal decision-making perspective. This broad perspective is required for several reasons. First, an agreed perspective cannot be the viewpoint of any single (set of) decision-maker(s), but should transcend individual interests – so it must be societal. Second, it cannot be based on current and geographically-specific institutional arrangements. For example, the perspective of the health care system will change over time (as the boundaries of what activities are regarded as health care develop) and would be specific to a national or regional system, but a societal decision-making perspective subsumes other narrower perspectives. Indeed, once an analysis is completed from the broadest perspective, it is possible to present the same analysis from the viewpoint of particular decision-makers.

It should be apparent, however, that an evaluation conducted from this broad societal perspective may not be directly relevant to specific stakeholders in the health care system who may have different objectives and constraints. Therefore, it should not be surprising if evaluations from a broad perspective have limited impact on actual decisions at 'lower levels' within the health care system, and which may suggest some institutional and managerial failure that could be addressed. The narrower perspective of particular decision-makers may be directly relevant to them, but can simply justify inefficient allocations without challenging existing institutional arrangements and incentives.

In common with many useful concepts, although the notion of a societal decision-maker is a useful concept, it is an abstraction. In the absence of a palpable Leviathan it seems useful to look to those institutions which have been given the remit, and therefore some form of legitimacy, to make societal decisions about health care (e.g. NICE in the UK). This does not imply that analysts must only reflect the concerns of these institutions (e.g. the NICE reference case for evaluation methods 2003); they also have a duty to point out the consequences of decisions for other groups of individuals and sectors of the economy. Although the full characterization of a legitimate societal decision-maker remains to be established, the advantage of a societal decision-making approach is that the basis and legitimacy of any normative prescriptions it makes are explicit and, therefore, open to debate. This contrasts sharply with the Welfarist approach where these are hidden behind notions of efficiency and remain implicit in the neoclassical view of the world.

Requirements for economic evaluation to inform decisions

If the societal decision-making paradigm is accepted as a valid theoretical foundation for economic evaluation, a series of requirements follow. In order to understand recent achievements and future challenges in this field, it is helpful to briefly summarize these:

- *Defining the decision problem.* The need for a clear statement of the relevant interventions and the groups of recipients. With respect to defining options, this will be all relevant and feasible options for the management of the recipient group.
- *The appropriate time horizon.* From a normative standpoint, it is clear how the time horizon of an analysis should be determined: it is the period over which the options under comparison are likely to differ in terms of costs and/or benefits. For any intervention that may have a plausible effect on mortality, this will require a lifetime time horizon to quantify the differential impact on life expectancy of the options under comparison.
- *Perspective on costs.* As discussed above, from a normative standpoint the argument for a societal perspective on costs is a strong one (Johannesson and O'Conor 1997), emphasizing the importance of avoiding externalizing resource costs on individuals and organizations outside of the direct focus of the decision-maker.
- *The objective function.* As argued above, there is no consensus on a legitimate objective function for purposes of societal decision-making. In the context of health care, however, systems are charged with improving the health of a given population. It follows, therefore, that the objective function in an economic evaluation seeking to inform decision-makers in this context would be based on some measure of health gain. A range of options exists regarding the exact definition of such a function – in particular, the source and specification of the preferences which determine its coefficients. The QALY has become widely used for this purpose, despite the strong assumptions necessary to link it to individual preferences (Pliskin *et al.* 1980).
- *Using available evidence.* For purposes of societal decision-making, economic evaluation needs to be able to use available evidence, allowing for its imperfections, to identify whether a technology is *expected* to be more cost-effective than its comparators – that is, it has higher *mean* cost-effectiveness. Moreover, the analysis needs to quantify the associated decision uncertainty which indicates the likelihood that, in deciding to fund a particular intervention,

the decision-maker is making the wrong decision. This provides a link to estimating the cost of decision uncertainty which, through value of information analysis, offers a basis for prioritizing future research.

RECENT ADVANCES IN ECONOMIC EVALUATION

A range of methods challenges is raised by these requirements. How far has economic evaluation come in the last ten years in meeting these challenges?

An analytical framework

Cost-effectiveness versus cost-benefit analysis

It is argued above that, within a societal decision-making paradigm in the field of health care, the objective function would be expected to be some measure of health gain. Valuing changes in health can be achieved using both CEA based on a generic measure of health such as a QALY or a healthy-year equivalent, or using cost-benefit analysis (CBA) based on monetary valuation derived using, for example, contingent valuation methods.

Methods research has recently been undertaken on both approaches to valuing health gain. However, it seems reasonable to argue that CEA should continue to be the type of study which predominates in economic evaluation in health care. First, the focus on health gain within the objective function in economic evaluation removes one of the putative advantages of contingent valuation – that is, the ability to value a range of health and non-health consequences of health care, where the latter might include attributes such as information and convenience. If these 'process' characteristics are not directly relevant in the objective function, then the choice between contingent valuation and non-monetary approaches comes down to which is more able to provide a reliable valuation of changes in health. Although this question is far from having been conclusively answered, the strength of CEA is that there has been more extensive use of non-monetary approaches to valuation. Second, CBA is founded on welfare economic theory, in particular the principle of the potential Pareto improvement as manifested in the compensation test (Sugden and Williams 1979). The rejection of these principles through the framework of societal decision-making suggests a rejection of CBA. The third reason for the focus on CEA is that, within the context of decision-making under a budget constraint, demonstrating a positive net benefit in a CBA is an insufficient basis to fund an intervention because, as for CEA, the opportunity cost of that decision on existing programmes needs to be quantified.

Trials versus models: the false dichotomy

For much of the period during which cost-effectiveness was developing a more prominent role in health care, there have been two parallel streams of applied work – that based on randomized trials and that centred on decision analytic models. Some authors have questioned the use of the decision model as a vehicle for economic evaluation (Sheldon 1996), being concerned about particular features such as the need to make assumptions. This literature has explicitly, or by implication, indicated a preference for trial-based cost-effectiveness analysis (CEA) where patient-level data are available on all relevant parameters. More recently, however, there has been a growing realization that trials and models are not alternative vehicles for economic evaluation, but are complementary (Claxton *et al.* 2002). This observation stems largely from the realization that the ultimate purpose of economic evaluation is to inform actual decision problems in a consistent manner based on an explicit definition of an objective function and constraints. Given this general requirement, it is clear that trials and decision models are doing quite different things. The purpose of randomized trials (or any primary study generating patient-level data) is to estimate particular parameters associated with a disease or the effects of health care interventions. The decision model, on the other hand, provides an analytical framework, based on explicit structural assumptions, within which available evidence can be combined and brought to bear on a clearly specified decision problem.

The realization that models and trials are not alternative analytical frameworks, and actually play different roles in the evaluation process, may be considered an achievement in its own right. There have, however, been some contributions to the methods of decision modelling. These include the role of such methods in characterizing uncertainty and informing research priorities. In addition, important work has covered the quality assessment of decision models for cost-effectiveness analysis (CEA) (Sculpher *et al.* 2000) and the need to link decision models to broader approaches to evidence synthesis (Cooper *et al.* in press).

Generating appropriate evidence

It is clear that the appropriate identification, measurement, analysis and synthesis of available evidence is an essential part of economic evaluation prior to incorporating these data into a decision model. Here 'evidence' refers to estimates of parameters such as absolute and relative treatment effects, HRQL, resource use and unit costs. The requirements for economic evaluation to support societal decision-making have some clear implications for evidence generation. These include the need to use all available evidence relating to an intervention and to estimate the mean value of parameters together with a relevant measure of uncertainty.

Analysis of patient-level data

Arguably, some of the most important achievements of the last decade in economic evaluation relate to the analysis of patient-level data. Most of these relate to statistical analysis for economic evaluation and, in particular, the appropriate quantification of uncertainty in individual parameters and in measures of cost-effectiveness analysis (CEA). The first of these is considered here, and the second is discussed more generally in the section below. A large proportion of this work has been undertaken in the context of trial-based economic evaluation, but its relevance extends to the analysis of observational data.

Skewed cost data
At first sight, the methods used to estimate the mean of a parameter would seem straightforward. However, the features of many patient-level data, particularly those relating to resource use and cost, complicate this process. One of these features is the positive skewness of the resource use and cost data which results from the fact that these measures are always positive but have no strict upper bound. The use of the median to summarize such distributions is unhelpful in economic evaluation because of the need to be able to link the summary measure of per patient cost to the total budget impact (Briggs and Gray 1998). Important work has been undertaken to reaffirm the focus on the mean and to provide a series of options in calculating its precision. These not only include the use of non-parametric bootstrapping (Briggs *et al.* 1997) and more detailed parametric modelling of individual resource use components (Cooper *et al.* 2003), but also the clarification that calculating

standard errors assuming a normal distribution is likely to be robust to skewness for reasonably large sample sizes (Briggs and Gray 1999).

Censored and missing data

The presence of censored data also complicates the process of estimating mean values with appropriate measures of dispersion. The most frequent example of this problem is when patients are entered into a trial at different time points, but follow-up is stopped – or analysis is undertaken – at a fixed moment in time. This results in costs which are derived from periods of follow-up which differ between patients, where this is not due to death but to the way the study is administered. An important contribution was to identify that taking a simple mean of available cost data in the presence of censoring will lead to biased estimates (Fenn *et al.* 1995). Subsequently, a range of methods has emerged in the literature which seeks to estimate mean cost while allowing for censoring under the assumption that non-censored patients are entirely representative of those who are censored. These methods started within a univariate statistical framework (Lin *et al.* 1997), but have since developed to include covariate adjustment (Lin 2000).

Censored data are a special case of the more general issue of missing data. A range of missing data problems has to be faced in most patient-level datasets used in economic evaluation. These include single items not being completed in case record forms or questionnaires, entire questionnaires being missing due to non-response and loss to follow-up where all data beyond a particular point are missing. A range of methods is available to cope with these various types of missing data, all of which require specific assumptions about the nature of the missing data but, unlike the techniques to cope with censored cost data, the development of these methods has not been specific to economic analysis (Briggs *et al.* 2003).

Multi-variable analysis

Until recently, regression analysis has played little role in economic evaluation. However, the rapid development of statistical methods in this field has included the realization that multi-variable analysis of patient-level data offers some major advantages for cost-effectiveness analysis (CEA). First, it gives scope to control for any imbalance between treatment groups in patients' baseline characteristics. Second, by controlling for prognostic baseline covariates, it provides more precise estimates of relevant treatment effects. Third, by facilitating estimates of the interaction between treatment undergone and baseline covariates, it provides an opportunity for subgroup analysis. As for univariate statistical analysis, important work has been undertaken in order to look at how the particular features of resource use and cost data can be appropriately analysed with regression. This has included the use of generalized linear models as a way of overcoming the heavy skewness in cost data referred to above, and the use of two-part models to deal with the fact that, for some interventions, a large proportion of patients incur zero costs (Lipscomb *et al.* 1996).

More recently, the use of regression analysis to analyse cost-effectiveness (rather than just cost) data has been considered, with the potential for use in the analysis of trial or observational data (Hoch *et al.* 2002). In part, this has been facilitated by the placement of cost-effectiveness onto a single scale using net benefits (Phelps and Mushlin 1991), where measures of outcome are valued in monetary terms on the basis of some form of threshold, willingness to pay measure. For the analysis of patient-level cost-effectiveness data, the independent variable becomes a patient-specific measure of net benefit.

The development of multi-variable methods has opened a range of analytical opportunities in economic evaluation relating to the modelling of variability. At its simplest, this involves the use of fixed effect models to adjust for patient-level covariates. Within the context of studies undertaken in multiple locations (e.g. the multi-centre and/or multi-national randomized trial), the use of multi-level modelling provides a means of assessing the variability in cost-effectiveness between locations (Sculpher *et al.* in press). Given the expectation that, due to factors such as variation in unit costs, epidemiology and clinical practice, costs and/or outcomes will vary by location, this type of analysis provides a means of considering the generalizability of economic evaluation results between locations.

Bayesian statistical methods
It has been argued above that statistical analysis has been one of the major areas of achievement in economic evaluation over the last decade. Much of this work, however, has involved applying methods developed outside economic evaluation to the analysis of cost-effectiveness data. A corollary of this is that some recent developments in statistics have benefited those undertaking cost-effectiveness analysis (CEA). Perhaps the best example of this is the development of Bayesian statistical methods in health care evaluation in general. This is largely a result of increased computer

power which facilitates the use of simulation methods where analytical approaches proved intractable (Spiegelhalter *et al.* 2003).

Bayesian approaches have proved valuable in economic evaluation for several reasons. First, the decision theoretic aspect of these methods has traditionally been an important element of economic evaluation in health care because decision analytic models are essentially Bayesian. The second advantage relates to the probability statements made possible using Bayesian approaches. That is, the ability to be able to present results which state the probability that a particular intervention is cost-effective given available evidence (i.e. decision uncertainty) is potentially more helpful to decision-makers than classical statistical analyses focused on standard rules of inference. Third, a major advantage of Bayesian statistics is the ability to bring to bear prior evidence in analysing new information. This is valuable for cost-effectiveness because it is consistent with the iterative approach to technology assessment (Fenwick *et al.* 2000b) whereby the cost-effectiveness of a given intervention is assessed based on existing evidence; the value (and optimal design) of additional research is based on decision uncertainty and the loss function in terms of health and resource costs; and, as new research is undertaken, it is used to update the priors and the iterative process begins again. Bayesian statistical methods have made an important contribution to the methods of synthesizing summary evidence. They have also had an impact on the analysis of patient-level data – for example, in relation to the modelling of costs (Cooper *et al.* 2003), and handling missing data (Lambert *et al.* 2003).

Analysis of summary data

Patient-level datasets provide important inputs into economic evaluation. In part, this relates to studies such as randomized trials which provide a possible vehicle for economic analysis. It has been argued, however, that most economic evaluations will involve the need to incorporate data from a range of sources. These will include patient-level datasets such as trials and observational studies, and the methods discussed above remain highly relevant to analyses of these data. A large proportion of the evidence needed for cost-effectiveness analysis (CEA) is, however, drawn from secondary sources where data are presented in summary form. There have been important developments in the synthesis and analysis of these data which, although they originate largely from statisticians, have considerable potential in economic evaluation. This potential stems from some of the requirements of economic evaluation described above: the need to use all available evidence and to characterize the uncertainty in parameters fully.

The process of synthesizing summary data could be achieved relatively straightforwardly, using methods like fixed effects meta-analysis, if the studies available in the literature directly compared the options of interest in the economic study; were all undertaken in the same sorts of patients treated with similar clinical practice; measured the same outcome measures; and reported at the same points of follow-up. In reality, the evidence base available for most cost-effectiveness studies is more complex than this, exhibiting many forms of heterogeneity, and this has necessitated the use of more sophisticated methods of synthesis. For purposes of cost-effectiveness, perhaps the greatest contribution has come from the use of Bayesian hierarchical modelling (Spiegelhalter *et al.* 2003). A major advantage of these techniques is that they provide parameter estimates (e.g. relative treatment effects) in the form necessary to provide the inputs into probabilistic decision models – that is, as random variables. Furthermore, this parameter uncertainty reflects not only their precision, but also the degree of heterogeneity between the data sources which, together with the uncertainty associated with all the other parameters, can be translated into decision uncertainty within the model.

One area where Bayesian hierarchical modelling has been used in evidence synthesis is to deal with situations where a series of options is being evaluated against each other but where direct head-to-head trial data do not exist. Indirect comparisons exist when the various options of interest have each been assessed within trials against a common option. This provides a conduit through which the absolute effects of all options can be compared. The more general situation has been termed 'mixed comparisons' where there is no common comparator but a network of evidence exists which links the effects of different options (e.g. trials of options A vs. C, D vs. E, A vs. E and D vs. C can be used as a basis for comparing all the options). Bayesian methods to generate parameter estimates, together with full measures of uncertainty in these contexts have been developed (Higgins and Whitehead 1996; Ades 2002). They have also been used in economic evaluations for NICE decision-making where lack of head-to-head trial data are more the rule than the exception.

Methods have also been developed to overcome other limitations in evidence. These include approaches to estimate a specific outcome based on data from all available trials, although it is measured in only a proportion of studies (Domenici *et al.* 1999); to estimate the relationship between an intermediate and final outcome measure using all available evidence on that link (Ades 2003); and to estimate a treatment effect at a particular point in follow-up using all trial data despite the fact that not all trials report at that time (Abrams *et al.* 2003). Although these methods have not yet been extensively used in economic evaluation, they are likely to provide important contributions in the future.

Cost data

Arguably, the generation of evidence from which unit costs can be estimated is one area where there have been few major contributions over the last few years. This is probably due to the modest resources invested in generating cost data compared to those devoted to gathering evidence on effectiveness and, increasingly, resource use. Although there are exceptions to this, particularly in the area of community-based services (Netten *et al.* 2000), economic evaluation in the National Health Service (NHS) continues to rely largely on evidence from imperfect routine sources such as the NHS Reference Costs (NHS Executive 2002), which show considerable variability in costing methods. Like other limitations in the available evidence base, this generates an additional source of uncertainty in cost-effectiveness analysis (CEA). It is important to characterize this source of uncertainty adequately given that economic theory would suggest an inter-relationship between unit costs (prices) and resource use (Raikou *et al.* 2000). However, the absence of sample data for unit costs means that little work has been undertaken to quantify this uncertainty using statistical methods. Rather, standard sensitivity analysis remains the main tool to investigate the extent to which uncertainty in unit costs impacts on the results of an analysis.

Applied cost-effectiveness analysis (CEA) continues to struggle with the reality of available unit cost data, at least in the NHS, but there have been some important areas of conceptual development in cost analysis, although the availability of data limits their application. Important work has been undertaken, for example, in considering the role of future costs in economic evaluation (Meltzer 1997). Perhaps the area generating the most literature in costing methods relates to productivity costs (Sculpher 2001). Initially stimulated by the deliberations and recommendations of the

Washington Panel (Gold *et al.* 1996), there has been valuable debate about the role of productivity costs in economic evaluation (Olsen 1994), the extent to which they are, or should be, reflected in the valuation of health rather than in monetary terms as 'costs' (Brouwer *et al.* 1997; Weinstein *et al.* 1997) and the duration over which productivity costs are relevant (Koopmanschap *et al.* 1995). Although productivity costs should probably have some role within a societal decision-making perspective, specific decision-makers vary in their attitude to the inclusion of these costs in studies (Hjelmgren *et al.* 2001).

Valuing health effects

Unlike the area of resource use, considerable research activity continues on methods and data used to value health effects within cost-effectiveness analysis (CEA). Some of this material is discussed in other chapters of this book, and the focus here is on two important areas of research. The first is the development, and increasingly widespread use, of generic preference-based measures of health status (Brazier *et al.* 1999). Their use in prospective studies has provided a valuable source of evidence, the features of which are consistent with the requirements described in the sections above. These are, namely, the focus on health effects and the use of a generic descriptive system to facilitate comparison between disease and technology areas. The last decade has seen the emergence of a number of validated descriptive systems, together with choice-based values based on samples of the public (Brazier *et al.* 1999). Further research is necessary to compare and contrast these instruments, with a view to undertaking some form of calibration or developing a synthesized measure including the strengths of each.

The second area of work to comment on here is the conceptual research associated with the QALY. Although the QALY has become an established measure of health benefit for cost-effectiveness analysis (CEA), there has been no shortage of literature detailing the strong assumptions under which the QALY would represent individual preferences (Pliskin *et al.* 1980; Loomes and McKenzie 1989). There have also been important contributions in the literature regarding possible alternatives to the QALY that are designed to reflect individuals' preferences about health effects more closely. Although, arguably, disproportionate attention has been paid in the literature to the relative merits and similarities between the measurement techniques, the healthy-years equivalent (HYE) represents an important development in the field, at least because it clarifies the QALY's assumptions regarding individuals' preferences over sequences of health states and prognoses (Mehrez and Gafni 1989). The development of the patient trade-off method also emphasized the mismatch between the typical derivation of a QALY based on an individual's valuation of health effects that they imagine experiencing themselves, and the ultimate social use of the measure in terms of allocating resources between individuals within a population context (Nord 1995). Related to this, there has also been valuable research on methods to incorporate individuals' equity preferences regarding health in a measure of benefit (Williams 1997; Nord *et al.* 1999).

Although the importance of this conceptual literature should not be underestimated, there has been very little use of these improvements on 'the simple QALY' in applied cost-effectiveness analysis (CEA). In part, this is likely to have been due to the additional demands they make in terms of measurement – this would certainly seem to be the case with the HYE. However, the failure of these developments of the QALY to take root in the applied cost-effectiveness literature may also reflect the lack of consensus about the appropriate objective function. For example, in order to allow for a more complex objective function regarding equity in health, more information is needed about social preferences concerning the trade-off between health gain and the features of the recipient.

Representing uncertainty in economic evaluation

We have summarized some of the important developments in statistical methods associated with the analysis of patient-level data. In part, this work has focused on appropriate estimation of particular parameters, including quantifying uncertainty. This is the case, for example, with the work on analysing missing and censored cost data. However, the most intellectual effort has gone into developing ways of calculating measures of dispersion around incremental cost-effectiveness. This can be seen as the process of translating parameter uncertainty in economic evaluation into decision uncertainty – that is, the likelihood that a particular option under evaluation is more cost-effective than its comparator(s).

Much of the research in this area has been concerned with the analysis of sampled patient-level data which provide direct estimates of treatment-specific mean costs and health effects together with measures of dispersion. In part, this work has considered ways of measuring the uncertainty around incremental cost-effectiveness ratios (ICERs) which are not straightforward, given, for example, the correlation between the numerator and denominator of these statistics. Important contributions include the rediscovery of statistical methods, such as Feiller's Theorem, to calculate confidence intervals around an ICER (Willan and O'Brien 1996) and the use of net benefits as a way of presenting cost-effectiveness and its uncertainty (Phelps and Mushlin 1991; Stinnett and Mullahy 1998).

An important area of work has also been to address the normative question of how uncertainty should be dealt with in making decisions about resource allocation. One perspective on this has been to reject the standard rules of inference reflected in the fixed error probabilities of the hypothesis test or the confidence interval (Claxton 1999). A strand of this argument is that the uncertainty around mean cost-effectiveness is irrelevant to the decision about which intervention to fund. This is because the objective of maximizing health outcome from finite resources requires a focus on expected (i.e. mean) costs and outcome, with the uncertainty around these means informing priorities about future research (Claxton 1999). This may be an area where the requirements of societal decision-making conflict with the specific incentives facing a particular decision-maker. Again, the role of economic analysis, within a societal decision-making paradigm, is to make those conflicts explicit by indicating the implications of decisions based on criteria other than expected cost-effectiveness.

Part of the process is to be clear about the decision uncertainty involved. That is, rather than present confidence intervals around an ICER, or a p-value for a null hypothesis of no difference in mean net benefit between alternative options, the decision-maker is presented with the probability that each of the options being compared is the most cost-effective given the decision-maker's maximum willingness to pay for a unit gain in health. These decision uncertainties are typically presented using cost-effectiveness acceptability curves (CEACs) which were initially developed to present uncertainty in patient-level data (Van Hout *et al.* 1994), but which are now fundamental to decision analytic models (Fenwick *et al.* 2001). Although these curves require the decision-maker to be clear about the value they attach to a unit gain in health, this was always the case in the interpretation of cost-effectiveness data.

CEACs are now routinely presented in trial-based cost-effectiveness studies (UK Prospective Diabetes Study Group 1998) and models (Chilcott *et al.* 2003). Their use as a way of presenting decision uncertainty in decision models results from another important development in cost-effectiveness analysis (CEA) in recent years: the use of probabilistic sensitivity analysis in models (Briggs *et al.* 2002). Until recently, cost-effectiveness analysis (CEA) based on decision models was only able to show the implications of parameter uncertainty using sensitivity analysis where a small number of parameters was varied over an arbitrary range, and the impact on the results was investigated. Given the large number of parameters in most decision models, this process was also seen as being partial. Probabilistic sensitivity analysis allows all parameters to be characterized as random variables – that is, as probability distributions rather than point estimates. Using Monte Carlo simulation, these multiple sources of parameter uncertainty are 'propagated' through the model and reflected as decision uncertainty using CEACs. Although there will always need to be a role for standard sensitivity (or scenario) analysis to look at the implications of uncertainty in, for example, model structure, probabilistic sensitivity analysis moves cost-effectiveness analysis (CEA) closer to the full characterization of parameter uncertainty. It should also be emphasized that, given that most decision models are non-linear, the correct way of estimating expected cost-effectiveness is through the use of probabilistic methods.

Informing research decisions

As argued in the last section, if the objective underlying the appraisal of health technologies is to make decisions that are consistent with maximizing health gains from available resources for all patients, then the adoption decision should be based on the expected (mean) cost-effectiveness of the technology given the existing information (Claxton 1999). However, this does not mean that adoption decisions can simply be based on little or poor quality evidence, as long as the decision to conduct further research to support adoption (or rejection) is made simultaneously.

A decision to adopt a technology based on existing information will be uncertain, and there will always be a chance that the wrong decision has been made, in which case costs will be incurred in terms of health benefit forgone. Therefore, the expected cost of uncertainty is determined jointly by the probability that a decision based on existing information will be wrong and the consequences of a wrong decision. Information is valuable because it reduces the chance of making the wrong decision and, therefore, reduces the expected costs of uncertainty surrounding the decision. The expected costs of uncertainty can be interpreted as the expected value of *perfect* information (EVPI) (Claxton and Posnett 1996). This is also the maximum that the health care system should be willing to pay for additional evidence to inform this decision in the future, and it places an upper bound on the value of conducting further research. These methods can be used to identify those clinical decision problems which should be regarded as priorities for further research. The value of reducing the uncertainty surrounding each of the input parameters in the decision model can also be established. In some circumstances, this will indicate which endpoints should be included in further experimental research, whilst, in others, it may focus research on getting more precise estimates of particular inputs which may not necessarily require experimental design and can be provided relatively quickly.

Expected value of information analysis has a firm foundation in statistical decision theory (Raiffa and Schlaifer 1959) and has been applied in other areas of research (Thompson and Evans 1997). However, important work in the field of health technology assessment has emerged over the last few years. Initially, this work was outlined using analytical solutions, which required assumptions of normally distributed data (Claxton 1998, 1999). Some of the implications of this type of analysis for an efficient regulatory framework for health technologies were demonstrated using stylized examples (Claxton 1998; Claxton *et al.* 2002). Until recently there have only been a few published applications to more complex decision analytic models (Fenwick *et al.* 2000b; Claxton *et al.* 2001). However, in recent years, non-parametric approaches to establishing EVPI and EVPI for model parameters have been clarified (Ades *et al.* forthcoming), and a number of applications to more complex decision models have been presented (Fenwick *et al.* 2000a; Claxton *et al.* 2003; Ginnelly *et al.* 2003).

This type of analysis can also inform the design of proposed research. It has been recognized for some time that it would be appropriate to base decisions about the design of research (optimal sample size, follow-up period and appropriate endpoints in a clinical trial) on explicit estimates of the additional benefits of the sample information and the additional costs (Berry 1993). This approach offers a number of advantages over more traditional approaches, which are based on the selection of an effect size which is worth detecting at traditional (and arbitrary) levels of statistical significance and power. Expected value of information theory offers a framework that can identify the expected value of sample information (EVSI) defined as the reduction in the expected cost of uncertainty surrounding the decision to adopt a technology as sample size increases. These expected benefits of sampling can be compared to expected costs to decide whether more sample information is worthwhile. This framework offers a means of ensuring that research designs are technically efficient in the sense that sample size, allocation of trial entrants, follow-up periods and the choice of endpoints are consistent with the objectives and the budget for the provision of health care.

Initially this framework for efficient research design used analytic solutions requiring assumptions of normality applied to simple stylized examples (Claxton 1998, 1999). These analytic solutions were also used to demonstrate that EVSI may have a useful application in the design of clinical research including sequential trial designs (Claxton *et al.* 2000), and in the selection of clinical strategies which should be included in proposed research (Claxton and Thompson 2001). More recently, methods to establish EVSI for a range of different types of model parameters without assuming normality of net benefit have been established (Ades *et al.* forthcoming).

METHODOLOGICAL CHALLENGES IN ECONOMIC EVALUATION

The foregoing sections of this chapter have attempted to make clear the important developments in the field of economic evaluation, but they also show the not inconsiderable areas of weakness in the methods as currently applied. These limitations have been highlighted by considering the demands of the societal decision-making perspective, in particular the need for a legitimate objective function and set of constraints. An important area of research in the field relates to the principles and practice of defining a legitimate objective function. Research challenges in this area include how a generic measure of health benefit can more accurately reflect individual preferences about health and the appropriate elicitation of social preferences regarding the equity of health care programmes, in particular which characteristics of the recipients of health gain should be taken into account in economic evaluation, and how trade-offs between efficiency and equity are to be quantified for this purpose. Other chapters in this book deal with this area in more detail.

Methods challenges also exist in areas which have traditionally been considered the remit of statistics and clinical epidemiology, such as the methods of evidence synthesis. These techniques are as much part of the process of evaluating the cost-effectiveness of an intervention as reflecting time preference through discounting. The process of incorporating all available evidence into a CEA, whilst reflecting all its uncertainties and heterogeneity, represents a key area of research activity over the next five years. This is particularly the case given the need for decision-makers to be more transparent regarding how they reach decisions. Notwithstanding the importance of research into the objective function and evidence synthesis, as well as a range of other conceptual and practical questions, here we focus on two particular areas for future methods research – more adequately dealing with the constraints in societal decision-making and the methods of research prioritization and design.

Constrained maximization

We have argued that the societal decision-making perspective involves maximizing a societal objective function subject to an exogenous budget constraint for health care. As currently operated, however, the budget constraint is rarely made explicit in cost-effectiveness studies. Rather, the cost-effectiveness of a new technology which requires more of the available budget than currently funded comparators, but generates additional health gain (i.e. it has a positive ICER), is typically assessed against an administrative rule of thumb about the system's willingness to pay for an additional unit of health. As has frequently been pointed out in the literature (Birch and Gafni 1992, 2002), this approach to decision-making fails to quantify the opportunity cost of the new programme. That is, within a budget constrained system, the opportunity cost of a new, more costly, programme is the intervention(s) which is/are displaced or down-scaled to fund it – the shadow price of the budget constraint. In systems without a binding budget constraint, the use of an arbitrary threshold, rather than explicitly considering opportunity cost, will inevitably lead to increases in health care expenditure. In systems where the budget is tightly fixed, the use of a threshold can lead to a hidden process of removing or contracting existing programmes to fund the new intervention. It has been argued that this is the case with the NICE technology appraisal system, where decisions to recommend new technologies that are not explicit about their opportunity cost result in local decision-makers having to identify savings from existing programmes without formal evidence and analysis (Sculpher *et al.* 2001).

This failure to use the full tools of cost-effectiveness and, instead, relying on arbitrary administrative thresholds, is a result of the dearth of evidence about the costs and health effects of those interventions funded from current budgets. Hence, for decision-making authorities such as NICE, the identity of the marginal programme(s) currently receiving funding, and the quantification of their costs and benefits, which determines the shadow price of the budget constraint, is usually unknown and would, anyway, vary between localities and over time. In this context, a series of research questions presents itself. In part, this would include an extensive programme of applied evaluation of currently funded programmes. This would certainly be a major undertaking, not least because current system-level policy arrangements in many jurisdictions focus on *new* technologies, usually pharmaceuticals. Although NICE, for example, is unusual among reimbursement authorities in considering non-pharmaceutical technologies, its focus has been on new interventions. Explicit consideration of opportunity cost in CEA is, therefore, likely to need some changes in the policy environment to accompany the additional research. For example, agencies such as NICE could be given a more balanced portfolio of technologies to appraise which, in addition to important new interventions, would include existing programmes where there is a prima facie case for reduced investment.

In addition to this programme of further applied work, there are technical questions to be resolved if the opportunity costs of new technologies are to be more explicitly considered in CEA. Although the standard decision rules of CEA are well defined (Johannesson and Weinstein 1993), they are based on a series of strong assumptions, including constant returns to scale, the absence of indivisibilities, and certainty regarding the costs and effects of potentially displaced programmes. To relax these assumptions, and to reflect budget constraints adequately, it is necessary to move to a more formal framework of constrained maximization using methods such as integer or linear mathematical programming. Although the role of these methods in CEA has been discussed in principle (Stinnett and Paltiel 1996), there have been few applications in policy-relevant research where budgets are allocated across diseases and specialties. It is particularly important to develop these methods to reflect the uncertainty in the cost and health effects of treatments. One use of such methods would be to provide decision-makers with clear

information not only about the uncertainty regarding the cost-
effectiveness of a new treatment but also about the risk that, in
reimbursing it, the total budget will be breached. Given the importance of 'staying within budget' in the organization and incentiviza-
tion of health care systems, this information will be valuable for
decision-makers – for example, it will facilitate consideration of the
role of insurance to protect budgets.

Considering the research agenda associated with the methods of
constrained maximization raises questions about the relevant constraints to include in such analyses. This is because the use of formal
mathematical programming provides the opportunity to include a
whole range of constraints, not just the relevant budget. In reality,
the constraints faced in decision-making are much more complex
and include a number of budget and capacity constraints over time.
These methods may also provide an opportunity for a more explicit
approach to dealing with other types of constraints faced by particular decision-makers which reflect broader policy initiatives in the
system. Some of these constraints may relate directly to resources –
such as the need to avoid staff redundancies. Others may relate to
non-resource considerations, such as the need to reduce (or, at least,
to avoid an increase in) waiting lists. In principle, the optimum allocation of resources to new and existing interventions can be established given this full range of constraints, but research is needed into
how to elicit these constraints, and how to specify them within
models. The promise of this area of methods research is that it can
highlight the conflicts between a societal decision-making perspective and the viewpoint of a particular decision-maker. This can be
achieved because each constraint within these models has a shadow
price. This can indicate what is being forgone in terms of health
benefits by implementing administrative constraints, for example,
associated with waiting lists.

Methods of research prioritization and design

In recent years substantial progress has been made in demonstrating
that the traditional rules of inference are irrelevant to rational
decision-making from a societal decision-making perspective.
Substantial progress has also been made in clarifying appropriate
methods of analysis of the value of information and their application
to more complex and policy-relevant models of health technologies.
However, a number of important challenges remain. The estimates
of value of information require all the uncertainties in the model to

be appropriately characterized. Failure to do so may only have a minor impact on the mean cost and effect but will, in most cases, have a much more substantial one on the estimates of the value of information. Therefore, more formal and explicit analysis of uncertainty for value of information analysis exposes many issues which, in the past, have been avoided or only considered implicitly. These include accounting for potential bias, considering the exchangeability of different sources of evidence, synthesizing evidence to make indirect comparisons, and using all direct and indirect evidence to estimate model parameters. As we have discussed, these issues are not really challenges specific to value of information analysis, but the adoption of more formal and explicit methods does make the importance of an appropriate characterization of uncertainty very clear, and places a greater responsibility on the analyst not only to use an appropriate point estimate for model parameters but also to use appropriate distributions based on a synthesis of all the evidence available.

There are also a number of issues specific to value of information. The methods for estimating overall EVPI and EVPI associated with parameters are now well established. However, there are computational challenges for complex models which will continue to be addressed by using more efficient sampling, more flexible programming languages and estimation techniques for computationally expensive models (Oakley and O'Hagan 2002). There are other issues such as the uncertainty over appropriate effective lifetimes of technologies, and incorporating some assessment of future technological developments, as well as the impact on clinical practice of adoption and research decisions. It is also increasingly important to consider the exchangeability of additional information with other patient subgroups and between different clinical decision problems.

The fundamental methods for estimating EVSI using conjugate priors is well established, although implementing these methods for real and more complex examples will undoubtedly pose as yet unresolved issues, for example the interpretation of random effects in an EVSI framework. Also, the issue of correlation between model parameters poses some problems as information about one will provide information about other correlated parameters. As the more sophisticated methods of evidence synthesis become more frequently used, this issue will become increasingly common because synthesis generates correlation between the parameters of interest.

The computational challenges are much more substantial for

EVSI than EVPI, and the approximation of linear relationships using analytical methods such as Taylor series expansions will be useful (Ades *et al.* forthcoming). However, the really interesting possibility is considering all the dimensions of design space both within and between studies. This includes sample size, allocation of sample, endpoints included and follow-up for a particular study. These have been addressed using analytical methods but have yet to be fully explored using Monte Carlo sampling. An even more challenging issue, at least in terms of computation, is establishing an efficient portfolio of studies and the optimal sequence of research designs. Finally, when priors are not conjugate then, in principle, Monte Carlo sampling could be used to generate predicted posterior distributions for the EVSI calculation. However, this will put the computation task on the edge of what is currently tractable even for simple and stylized models.

CONCLUSIONS

The last decade has seen some major achievements in economic evaluation methods. These have largely related to technical methods associated with statistical analysis of patient-level data, usually alongside trials, the use of decision theory to evaluate interventions under uncertainty and to assist in research prioritization and the valuation of health within the QALY framework. It is not easy to judge the value of advances in methods unless there is clarity about the question that economic evaluation is seeking to address. This chapter argues in favour of a societal decision-making role for economic evaluation. Many of the methods developments in recent years are consistent with this perspective, but this view may not be shared by those who believe welfare economic theory should be the theoretical foundation upon which economic evaluation is based. There is, therefore, a need for further debate about the appropriate theoretical framework for this area of research.

Even if there is agreement about the value of a societal decision-making perspective, a large number of gaps in the methods of economic evaluation will have to be filled for this perspective to be fully realized in practice. Some of these gaps combine both conceptual and practical issues. An important example of this is how to define and elicit a legitimate objective function which reflects social preferences: although the measurement of benefit within a QALY framework has become more rigorous, this remains a crude characterization of a legitimate objective function. Many other gaps exist regarding the technical methods used to synthesize available evidence, characterize its uncertainty, design additional research and adequately reflect budget and other constraints. Many of these technical methods questions are not traditionally areas of interest for the economist, generating more excitement among statisticians, epidemiologists and operations researchers. However, this emphasizes the multi-disciplinary nature of cost-effectiveness research and the unavoidable conclusion that, for this research to be relevant to policy, it needs to be seen less as *economic* evaluation, and more as evaluation.

DISCUSSION
Trevor Sheldon

This chapter provides an excellent summary of recent developments and future challenges for economic evaluation methods in health care. It provides a clear description of the increasingly high-profile role these methods are playing in some areas of health care decision-making – particularly regarding the reimbursement of new pharmaceuticals. The NICE technology appraisal process in the UK perhaps provides the most stark example of a decision-making authority demanding formal economic analysis of new technologies based on a highly prescriptive definition of appropriate methods.

The authors provide a very positive perspective regarding how economic analysis can inform decision-making. In this discussion I would like to consider some of the issues that I see within the role and methods of economic evaluation in health care.

The first issue is that I think we have seen a major change in the links between economic evaluation and economic theory. As highlighted in the chapter, the methods increasingly used in the field probably owe more to the disciplines of statistics (particularly statistical decision theory) and operational research than to economics. There have undoubtedly been some important benefits from the movement away from mainstream economic theory. These include a greater attention to generating appropriate estimates of the effectiveness of health technologies as part of the process of assessing efficiency, and more focus on quantifying the uncertainty associated with cost-effectiveness. However, maybe there have been some downsides – for example, little attention seems to be paid to the methods and process of estimating the costs and cost implications of health technologies. The authors provide an interesting critique of welfare economic theory – the traditional theoretical foundation of economic appraisal – but I worry whether 'cutting the umbilical cord' with economics will leave economic evaluation in a 'theoretical limbo' dominated by techniques rather than anchored in a normative framework grounded in economic theory. Important research is therefore needed to develop further the societal decision-making viewpoint as a normative framework for decision-making. There would also be benefit from studying how other areas of applied economic evaluation (e.g. transport, environment) have handled the limitations of welfare theory. Is the same movement away from 'the mother discipline' evident in these areas?

A second issue relates to the measurement and valuation of health. Although this is dealt with as a specific area of research in other chapters, it remains an important element of economic evaluation more generally. I have some concerns about the scientific underpinnings of some of the measures which have been developed and are now routinely used in economic evaluation. I wonder whether the scientific development of these measures has been stunted by the tendency for many of the key researchers in this field to divide into 'camps' associated with particular benefit measures and instruments. The distinctions are often not explicitly based on fundamental differences in theoretical approaches or even techniques for eliciting valuations or analysis, but more on what people happen to have done or the historical context of instrument development, and are often perpetuated by national or institutional rivalries or even personal gain. I believe much more insight into appropriate methods in this key area would be achieved through full collaboration and a willingness to compare instruments and methods. The whole edifice of economic evaluation rests crucially on how health (and other relevant outcomes) are measured and valued, and I feel we have become too accepting of what is routinely available and commonly used, rather than continuing to strive for improved measures.

A third, and related, issue is whether economic evaluation focuses too greatly on health, rather than taking a broader view of benefits. This is discussed in the chapter, with a recognition that other arguments might appropriately enter the utility of a decision-making body. However, it is clear that, as currently practiced, most applied economic evaluations rarely extend their measures of outcome beyond those that are defined in terms of health. This obsession with health as opposed to the broader elements of welfare (possibly a consequence of the move away from welfare theory) has, I believe, some unfortunate implications. First, the constraint it places on analysis to inform appropriate health care budgets: recognizing the broader effects on societal welfare of the services delivered by health care would, at least, provide a more informed basis for policymakers' deliberations about budgets. Second, it feeds a disproportionate interest in *technologies* focused on disease, rather than programmes which encompass a broader view of how to improve individuals' welfare. Third, the exclusive focus on health outcomes (including HRQLs) reinforces society's increasing obsession with *health* and so health care, rather than overall *welfare*. This, in turn, helps justify increased spending on health care which, as we have seen in the USA, can reach absurd levels coexisting with poor levels of overall welfare. While this might be advantageous to health care providers and suppliers (as this ultimately increases their incomes), it is unlikely to be optimal for the public. A refocus on welfare (which may be difficult given the alienation from mainstream economics) would allow more sensible choices as to how much public spending should be and how this investment should be allocated.

The final issue I would like to raise relates to the role and objectives of the decision-making agencies which are now seeking to be informed by economic evaluation. Do these agencies really have an objective function centred on health gain or societal welfare, or is economic evaluation providing a flexible 'technical veneer' to justify decisions which are actually based on opaque political considerations? A second concern is the willingness of these agencies to accept the poor data which manufacturers often submit to them as a basis for making decisions. The importance of using methods, such as value of information analysis, as a basis to demand additional evidence is a significant contribution of the chapter. A third concern is that agencies such as NICE in the UK and the process they demand for submissions are, directly or indirectly, absorbing a large proportion of the available expertise in economic evaluation. Are there not more important questions which these researchers should be addressing than whether particular new drugs represent good value to the health system? Finally, I worry about the agencies' lack of consideration of the opportunity cost of their decisions. I agree with the authors that we need an analytical framework which more explicitly considers what health care systems have to give up to fund new technologies.

In summary, I believe this chapter clearly sets out the achievements of economic evaluation in health as well as the challenges. As acknowledged by the authors, the more that is achieved, the more we understand how far we still have to go.

REFERENCES

Abrams, K., Sutton, A., Cooper, N., Sculpher, M., Palmer, S., Ginnelly, L. and Robinson, M. (2003) Populating economic decision models using meta-analysis of heterogeneously reported studies augmented with expert beliefs. Paper presented at Developing Economic Evaluation Methods (DEEM) workshop, Bristol.

Ades, A. (2002) A chain of evidence with mixed comparisons: models for multi-parameter synthesis and consistency of evidence. Paper presented at the Developing Economic Evaluation Methods meeting, Oxford, April.

Ades, A.E. (2003) A chain of evidence with mixed comparisons: models for multi-parameter synthesis and consistency of evidence, *Statistics in Medicine*, 22: 2995–3016.

Ades, A.E., Lu, G. and Claxton, K. (forthcoming) Expected value of sample information in medical decision modelling, *Medical Decision Making*.

Arrow, K. and Scitovsky, T. (1969) *Readings in Welfare Eonomics*. London: Allen & Unwin.

Berry, D.A. (1993) A case for Bayesianism in clinical trials, *Statistics in Medicine*, 12: 1377–93.

Birch, S. and Gafni, A. (1992) Cost effectiveness/utility analyses: do current decision rules lead us to where we want to be? *Journal of Health Economics*, 11: 279–96.

Birch, S. and Gafni, A. (2002) On being NICE in the UK: guidelines for technology appraisal for the NHS in England and Wales, *Health Economics*, 11: 185–91.

Boadway, R.W. (1974) The welfare foundations of cost-benefits analysis, *Economic Journal*, 84: 96–9.

Brazier, J., Deverill, M., Green, C., Harper, R. and Booth, A. (1999) A review of the use of health status measures in economic evaluation, *Health Technology Assessment*, 3(9).

Briggs, A. and Gray, A. (1998) The distribution of health care costs and their statistical analysis for economic evaluation, *Journal of Health Services Research and Policy*, 3(4): 233–45.

Briggs, A.H. and Gray, A. (1999) Handling uncertainty when performing economic evaluation of health care interventions, *Health Technology Assessment*, 3.

Briggs, A.H., Wonderling, D.E. and Mooney, C.Z. (1997) Pulling cost-effectiveness analysis up by its bootstraps: a non-parametric approach to confidence interval estimation, *Health Economics*, 6: 327–40.

Briggs, A.H., Goeree, R., Blackhouse, G. and O'Brien, B.J. (2002) Probabilistic analysis of cost-effectiveness models: choosing between treatment strategies for gastroesophageal reflux disease, *Medical Decision Making*, 22: 290–308.

Briggs, A.H., Clark, T., Wolstenholme, J. and Clarke, P.M. (2003) Missing . . . presumed at random: cost-analysis of incomplete data, *Health Economics*, 12: 377–92.

Brouwer, W.B.F., Koopmanschap, M.A. and Rutten, F.F.H. (1997) Productivity costs measurement through quality of life? A response to the recommendation of the Washington Panel, *Health Economics*, 6: 253–9.

Chilcott, J., McCabe, C., Tappenden, P., O'Hagan, A., Cooper, N.J., Abrams, K. and Claxton, K. (on behalf of the Cost-Effectiveness of Multiple Sclerosis Therapies Study Group) (2003) Modelling the cost effectiveness of interferon beta and glatiramer acete in the management of multiple sclerosis, *British Medical Journal*, 326: 522.

Claxton, K. (1998) Bayesian approaches to the value of information: implications for the regulation of new pharmaceuticals, *Health Economics Letters*, 2: 22–8.

Claxton, K. (1999) The irrelevance of inference: a decision-making approach to the stochastic evaluation of health care technologies, *Journal of Health Economics*, 18: 342–64.

Claxton, K. and Posnett, J. (1996) An economic approach to clinical trial design and research priority-setting, *Health Economics*, 5: 513–24.

Claxton, K. and Thompson, K.A. (2001) Dynamic programming approach to efficient clinical trial design, *Journal of Health Economics*, 20: 432–48.

Claxton, K., Walker, S. and Lacey, L. (2000) Selecting treatments: a decision theoretic approach, *Journal of the Royal Statistical Society*, 163: 211–25.

Claxton, K., Neuman, P.J., Araki, S.S. and Weinstein, M.C. (2001) The value of information: an application to a policy model of Alzheimer's disease, *International Journal of Technology Assessment in Health Care*, 17: 38–55.

Claxton, K., Sculpher, M. and Drummond, M. (2002) A rational framework for decision-making by the National Institute for Clinical Excellence, *Lancet*, 360: 711–15.

Claxton, K., Sculpher, M.J., Palmer, S. and Philips, Z. (2003) The cost-effectiveness and value of information associated with repeat screening for age related macular degeneration (abstract), *Medical Decision Making*, 23: 6.

Cooper, N.J., Sutton, A.J., Mugford, M. and Abrams, K.R. (2003) Use of Bayesian Markov Chain Monte Carlo methods to model cost data, *Medical Decision Making*, 23: 38–53.

Cooper, N.J., Sutton, A.J., Abrams, K.R., Turner, D. and Wailoo, A. (in press) Comprehensive decision analytical modelling in economic evaluation: a Bayesian approach. *Health Economics.*

Domenici, F., Parmigiani, G., Wolpert, R.L. and Hasselblad, V. (1999) Meta-analysis of migraine headache treatments: combining information from heterogenous designs, *Journal of the Amercian Statistical Association*, 94: 16–128.

Duthie, T., Trueman, P., Chancellor, J. and Diez, L. (1999) Research into the use of health economics in decision-making in the United Kingdom – Phase II: is health economics 'for good or evil'? *Health Policy*, 46: 143–57.

Fenn, P., McGuire, A., Phillips, V., Backhouse, M. and Jones, D. (1995) The analysis of censored treatment cost data in economic evaluation, *Medical Care*, 33(8): 851–63.

Fenwick, E., Claxton, K. and Sculpher, M. (2000a) A Bayesian analysis of pre-operative optimisation of oxygen delivery (abstract), *Medical Decision Making*, 20: 4.

Fenwick, E., Claxton, K., Sculpher, M. and Briggs, A. (2000b) Improving the efficiency and relevance of health technology assessment: the role of decision analytic modelling. Centre for Health Economics Discussion Paper 179.

Fenwick, E., Claxton, K. and Sculpher, M. (2001) Representing uncertainty: the role of cost-effectiveness acceptability curves, *Health Economics*, 10: 779–89.

Garber, A.M. and Phelps, C.E. (1997) Economic foundations of cost-effectiveness analysis, *Journal of Health Economics*, 16: 1–31.

Ginnelly, L., Claxton, K., Sculpher, M.J. and Philips, Z. (2003) The cost-effectiveness and value of information associated with long-term antibiotic treatment for preventing recurrent urinary tract infections in children (abstract), *Medical Decision Making*, 23: 6.

Gold, M.R., Siegel, J.E., Russell, L.B. and Weinstein, M.C. (1996) *Cost-Effectiveness in Health and Medicine.* New York: Oxford University Press.

Green, J. (1976) *Consumer Theory.* London: Macmillan.

Grossman, M. (1972) On the concept of health capital and the demand for health, *Journal of Political Economy*, 80: 223–49.

Higgins, J.P.T. and Whitehead, J. (1996). Borrowing strength from external trials in meta-analysis, *Statistics in Medicine*, 15: 2733–49.

Hjelmgren, J., Berggren, F. and Andersson, F. (2001) Health economic guidelines – similarities, differences and some implications, *Value in Health*, 4(3): 225–50.

Hoch, J.S., Briggs, A.H. and Willan, A. (2002) Something old, something new, something borrowed, something BLUE: a framework for the marriage of health econometrics and cost-effectiveness analysis, *Health Economics*, 11(5): 415–30.

Johannesson, M. and O'Conor, R.M. (1997) Cost-utility analysis from a societal perspective, *Health Policy*, 39: 241–53.

Johannesson, M. and Weinstein, S. (1993) On the decision rules of cost-effectiveness analysis, *Journal of Health Economics*, 12: 459–67.

Koopmanschap, M.A., Rutten, F.F.H., van Ineveld, B.M. and van Roijen, L. (1995) The friction cost method of measuring the indirect costs of disease, *Journal of Health Economics*, 14: 123–262.

Lambert, P., Billingham, C., Cooper, N., Sutton, A.J. and Abrams, K.R. (2003) Estimating the cost-effectiveness of an intervention in a clinical trial when partial cost information is available: a Bayesian approach. Paper presented at Developing Economic Evaluation Methods (DEEM) workshop, Aberdeen.

Lin, D.Y. (2000) Linear regression analysis of censored medical costs, *Biostatistics*, 1: 35–47.

Lin, D.Y., Feuer, E.J., Etzioni, R. and Wax, Y. (1997) Estimating medical costs from incomplete follow-up data, *Biometrics*, 53: 419–34.

Lipscomb, J., Ancukiewicz, M., Parmigiani, G., Hasselblad, V., Samsa, G. and Matchar, D.B. (1996) Predicting the cost of illness: a comparison of alternative models applied to stroke, *Medical Decision Making*, 18 (supplement): S39–56.

Loomes, G. and McKenzie, L. (1989) The use of QALYs in health care decision-making, *Social Science and Medicine*, 28: 299–308.

Machina, M.J. (1987) Choice under uncertainty: problems solved and unsolved, *Economic Perspectives*, 1: 121–54.

Mehrez, A. and Gafni, A. (1989) *Healthy Years Equivalents: How to Measure them Using the Standard Gamble Approach.* Hamilton, Ontario: CHEPA, McMaster University.

Meltzer, D. (1997) Accounting for future costs in medical cost-effectiveness analysis, *Journal of Health Economics*, 16: 33–64.

Netten, A., Dennett, J. and Knight, J. (2000) *Unit Costs of Health and Social Care.* Canterbury: PSSRU, University of Kent.

Ng, Y.K. (1983) *Welfare Economics: Introduction and Development of Basic Concepts.* London: Macmillan.

NHS Executive (2002) *The New NHS – 2002 Reference Cost.* London: NHS Executive, http://www.doh.gov.uk/nhsexec/refcosts.htm.

NICE (National Institute for Clinical Excellence) (2001) *Technical Guidance for Manufacturers and Sponsors on making a Submission to a Technology Appraisal*, http://www.nice.org.uk.

NICE (National Institute for Clinical Excellence) (2003) *Guide to the Methods of Technology Appraisal* (draft for consultation). London: NICE.

Nord, E. (1995) The person-tradeoff approach to valuing health care programs, *Medical Decision Making*, 15: 201–8.

Nord, E., Pinto, J.L., Richardson, J., Menzel, P. and Ubel, P. (1999) Incorporating societal concerns for fairness in numerical valuations of health programmes, *Health Economics*, 8: 25–39.

Oakley, J. and O'Hagan, A. (2002) Bayesian inference for the uncertainty distribution of computer model outputs, *Biometrika*, 89: 769–84.

Olsen, J.A. (1994) Production gains: should they count in health care evaluations? *Scottish Journal of Political Economy*, 41(1): 69–84.

Pauly, M.V. (1995) *Valuing Health Benefits in Monetary Terms*. Cambridge: Cambridge University Press.

Phelps, C.E. and Mushlin, A. (1991) On the near equivalence of cost-effectiveness analysis and cost-benefit analysis, *International Journal of Technology Assessment in Health Care*, 17: 12–21.

Pliskin, J.S., Shepard, D.S. and Weinstein, M.C. (1980) Utility functions for life years and health status, *Operations Research*, 28(1): 206–24.

Raiffa, H. and Schlaifer, R. (1959) *Probability and Statistics for Business Decisions*. New York: McGraw-Hill.

Raikou, M., Briggs, A., Gray, A. and McGuire, A. (2000) Centre-specific or average unit costs in multi-centre studies? Some theory and simulation, *Health Economics*, 9: 191–8.

Sculpher, M.J. (2001) The role and estimation of productivity costs in economic evaluation, in M.F. Drummond and A.E. McGuire (eds) *Theory and Practice of Economic Evaluation in Health*. Oxford: Oxford University Press.

Sculpher, M.J., Fenwick, E. and Claxton, K. (2000) Assessing quality in decision analytic cost-effectiveness models: a suggested framework and example of application, *Pharmacoeconomics*, 17(5): 461–77.

Sculpher, M.J., Drummond, M.F. and O'Brien, B.J. (2001) Effectiveness, efficiency, and NICE, *British Medical Journal*, 322: 943–4.

Sculpher, M.J., Pang, F. and Manca, A. (in press) Assessing the generalizability of economic evaluation studies, *Health Technology Assessment*.

Sheldon, T.A. (1996) Problems of using modelling in the economic evaluation of health care, *Health Economics*, 5: 1–11.

Spiegelhalter, D.J., Abrams, K.R. and Myles, J.P. (2003) *Bayesian Approaches to Clinical Trials and Health-care Evaluation*. London: Wiley.

Stinnett, A.A. and Mullahy, J. (1998) Net health benefits: a new framework for the analysis of uncertainty in cost-effectiveness analysis, *Medical Decision Making*, 18: S68–80.

Stinnett, A.A. and Paltiel, A.D. (1996) Mathematical programming for the efficient allocation of health care resources, *Journal of Health Economics*, 15: 641–53.

Sugden, R. and Williams, A.H. (1979) *The Principles of Practical Cost-Benefit Analysis*. Oxford: Oxford University Press.

Thompson, K.M. and Evans, J.S. (1997) The value of improved national exposure information for perchloroethylene (perc): a case study for dry cleaners, *Risk Analysis*, 17: 253–71.

UK Prospective Diabetes Study Group (1998) Cost effectiveness analysis of improved blood pressure control in hypertensive patients with type 2 diabetes: UKPDS 40, *British Medical Journal*, 317: 720–6.

Van Hout, B.A., Al, M.J., Gordon, G.S. and Rutten, F.F.H. (1994) Costs, effects and c/e-ratios alongside a clinical trial, *Health Economics*, 3: 309–19.

Weinstein, M.C. and Manning, W.G. (1997) Theoretical issues in cost-effectiveness analysis, *Journal of Health Economics*, 16: 121–8.

Weinstein, M.C., Siegel, J.E. and Garber, A.M. (1997) Productivity costs, time costs and health-related quality of life (HRQL): a response to the Erasmus group, *Health Economics*, 6; 505–10.

Willan, A. and O'Brien, B. (1996) Confidence intervals for cost-effectiveness ratios: an application of Fieller's Theorem, *Health Economics*, 5: 297–305.

Williams, A. (1997) Intergenerational equity: an exploration of the 'fair innings' argument, *Health Economics*, 6: 117–32.

2

VALUING HEALTH OUTCOMES: TEN QUESTIONS FOR THE INSOMNIAC HEALTH ECONOMIST

Paul Kind

INTRODUCTION

Fundamental to all economic evaluations of health care is the capacity to detect and quantify health outcomes, defined here as changes in health status over time. The past 30 years have seen the development of robust methods of measurement for use in this role. From simple measures based on mortality to more complex measures of health-related quality of life (HRQL), the impetus for improvement has arisen from the increasingly sophisticated demands of the health economist. However, despite their fundamental role, no general consensus has so far emerged as to the standards of design or performance that are required of outcome measures. While the methodological steps in instrument design and construction are well recognized, opinion remains divided as to a single standard mode of measurement. Measures of health status typically incorporate twin systems of description and valuation. A means of describing health status is a necessary prerequisite to its valuation. Health economics has acted as the driving force in shaping this latter aspect. Indeed, it is the increased demand for preference-based measures in economic evaluation that has fuelled much of the development of valuation of health. Progress has been remarkable in terms of the increased complexity and sophistication of the research field itself – issues such as 'states worse than dead' were not recognized three decades ago and are now part of the mainstream. However, there remain unresolved questions, and new challenges emerge as the environment in which the valuation agenda is contained expands.

Lest what follows be regarded as 'too pessimistic',[1] it is right to acknowledge the undoubted progress made in the field of health status measurement. Progress in terms of both concept and methods – from the conceptual beginnings of the early 1970s (Culyer *et al.* 1972) through to the formal investigation of health state valuations of the 1990s (Dolan *et al.* 1996). Progress in investigating values for health – from magnitude estimation (Rosser and Kind 1978) to Time Trade-Off (TTO) (Torrance *et al.* 1973) and Standard Gamble (SG) (Brazier *et al.* 2002). Progress in constructing instruments – from the Rosser Index (Rosser and Watts 1972) through to EQ-5D (Brooks 1996) and SF-6D (Brazier *et al.* 2002). There can be little doubt about the advancement of knowledge and the improvement in practice. However, the excellence of the research endeavour and the robustness of its product does not fully dispose of the larger context in which many issues remain unresolved – and, more troubling, sometimes unacknowledged.

Health economics can point to several important milestones in its brief existence. The quality-adjusted life year (QALY) can be identified in the literature prior to the early 1970s, but its emergence in the latter part of that decade provided health economists with an important unit of measure – and spun-off an almost separate research 'industry'. The Washington Panel (Gold *et al.* 1996) on the cost-effectiveness of medicine produced much needed guidance for the practicing health economist. For UK health economists or, more precisely, health economists who practise within England and Wales, the establishment of the National Institute for Clinical Excellence (NICE) was a further landmark event, irrevocably changing the environment within which economic evaluation operates and modifying the rules by which that evaluation is conducted. Similar institutions are to be found in other countries too (e.g. Australia and Canada). Guidance on the conduct of technology appraisals includes the stipulation that benefits should be expressed in terms of QALYs NICE 2004). The irresistible imperative to quantify the outcomes to health care interventions created by the convergence of these influential events presents a real dilemma for the health economist, both as the creator, and user, of the QALY technology. Not only is the range and complexity of issues related to this topic greater than was the case a decade ago, but we are yet to form a consensus about the way ahead. It is doubtful too, whether those who apply the QALY technology are always sufficiently well informed about its genesis, or sufficiently self-critical in their use of it. In short, the overwhelming need to compute a QALY suppresses the natural inclination of the health economist to probe and question the evidence base that confronts them. As a consequence, we risk damaging the credibility of the measurement technology through inappropriate usage. So long as the general public and other non-technocrats remain ignorant of the turmoil behind the technology, health economists have an opportunity to address some of the design issues that underpin the measurement of health outcomes. This chapter is intended as a contribution to that process – to help stimulate health economists to new activity today, or to enable them to sleep more peacefully with the promise of waking reinvigorated tomorrow.

VALUE AND VALUATION

Value and value judgement play a central role in all aspects of the planning, delivery and execution of health care. Sometimes, but rarely, those values are explicit. Sometimes they can be inferred. More generally, they remain concealed. It was once observed that health economics shines a light on the dark places inhabited by health care professionals. Nowhere should the light be brighter than in illuminating the process by which QALYs are computed, for here is *the* classic instance in which values are critical. Small differences in the denominator can have a disproportionate impact on a cost-effectiveness ratio. In making values explicit, any residual issues linked to the mechanism by which they are produced can also be rehearsed. Simply promulgating an explicit set of values is only half the story. It is rather like providing an inexperienced motorist with access to a high performance race vehicle. A minimum acquired level of knowledge, sophistication and maturity is needed to drive without risking the safety of all concerned. Simply offering up a social 'tariff'[2] and delegating the responsibility for working through the evidence of its genesis to the end-user is to deny the proper function of the research scientist.

MEASUREMENT DESIDERATA

The QALY is a scalar unit of measure that is the product of survival duration (measured in units of time) and a quality-adjustment factor (indicating the relative value of each time period). To fulfil this arithmetic role legitimately, the quality-adjustment factor must be of a single index form and (for practical reasons) that index must lie on a scale that assigns a value of 1 to full health and a value of 0 to dead. For the purposes of cost-utility analysis it is the general convention that the weight associated with all other health states is to be measured in terms of utility (or, more generally, as some measure of social value). The methods by which utilities are measured, and the source of those reference utilities, will be discussed later.

Technical advice published by NICE (2004), made recommendations for data intended for the measurement of benefit in cost-utility analysis. It called for 'a quality-adjustment index based on the preferences of the general public in England and Wales expressed as a cardinal measure of utility'. This encapsulates several intrinsic properties of the measurement instrument used in QALY computations. Table 2.1 sets out the principal attributes demanded of any quality-adjustment factor that might be considered for use in NICE appraisals. Some properties are more critical than others. For example, it would be inconceivable to undertake any arithmetic without access to a quality-adjustment factor that had an index format. Nor would it be acceptable were such a process conducted using a scale that lacked cardinal properties. These first three attributes are strictly non-negotiable and failure to conform with any of them should be regarded as an irrecoverable defect. There *may* be more scope for flexibility in respect of the last three attributes. Accepting an alternate definition of **relevant** population could lead to the recognition of, say, patient-based values or those generated in a non-UK population setting. Accepting preference elicitation methods that are *not* designed to generate utilities might be a further option.

Table 2.1 Attributes of a quality-adjustment factor

Intrinsic attributes of the instrument		Criticality	Scope for flexibility
A	Index format	XXXX	Nil
B	Cardinal scale	XXX	Nil
C	0 (dead) – 1 (full health) metric	XX	Nil
D	Weights derived from relevant population	X	Limited
E	Explicit preference-based weighting system	?	Limited
F	Generic descriptive system	?	Limited

METHODS OF ELICITATION

Measuring social preferences can be achieved using many different techniques, with the choice of method being largely driven by its intended application. In the context of decision analysis and economic evaluation or, more generally, where the concept of utility is the adopted model for representing such preferences, the set of candidate methods for eliciting preferences is limited. The measurement of utility consistent with the interpretation of von Neumann-Morgenstern axioms (von Neumann and Morgenstern 1944) suggests that SG should be the preferred method of elicitation. However, a less restrictive interpretation accepts other methods, which are based on the principle of sacrifice. Notable among such alternatives is TTO, proposed by Bush (Fanshel and Bush 1970) and Torrance (Torrance *et al.* 1973) as a means of generating weights for a health status measure that might be combined with data on survival to yield a quality-adjusted product. Quality-adjusted health status had coincidentally emerged elsewhere at the same time (Grogono and Woodgate 1971). The use of other methods, such as rating scales, and of data processing techniques, such as conjoint analysis, have added to the set of methods that might now be considered as potential approaches to the derivation of utility weights. There is a general resistance towards conjoint analysis although paradoxically health economists seem generally inclined to accept rating scales alongside SG and TTO as the basis of utilities. However, since weights based on rating scales typically avoid both uncertainty and exchange, it is hard to see the case for their use in a raw form as anything other than ordinal measures of utility. Analytic methods that enable cardinal scales to be derived from ordinal data have long been recognized in other disciplines. Paired comparisons methods (Thurstone 1927) are well suited to the construction of indifference curves but have only occasionally found favour in valuing health (Fanshel and Bush 1970; McKenna *et al.* 1981; Hadorn *et al.* 1992). The proximal needs of market research provide strong indications of other viable techniques suitable for use in establishing social preferences for health, such as multi-dimensional scaling(Green *et al.* [1970] 1989).

One might be tempted to make a case for preferring SG on the grounds of theory. Indeed, since the existence of a theory (any theory) seems to confer a mystical superiority on procedures designed to capture utilities, SG has a substantial advantage in this regard. The absence of an accessible theoretical base, by contrast, seems to condemn alternative procedures to the academic waste-lands. Supposing, however, for a moment, that there was theoretical 'blue water' that divided SG from other candidate techniques, then this would undermine the status of utilities estimated using non-SG methods. Although this might be an uncomfortable position for those who do not accept the claims for its superiority, such a move has the merit of simplifying the situation. SG becomes *the* method of choice.

An important issue is that the two principal methods of elicitation yield different estimates. Weights derived using SG are known to differ from corresponding weights derived using TTO. The reluctance to entertain even the smallest risk of death in order to forgo any portion of life expectancy at all, to avoid remaining in an apparently minor dysfunctional health state, is well known. In the face of such demonstrable failure of the nominated 'standard' tech-niques, researchers continue to struggle to reconcile the differences in empirical data generated using these methods. Were evidence avail-able that supported the dominance of SG, then the issue of valuation method might be settled beyond doubt. However, since the practical procedure of implementing SG is itself open to local interpretation[3] and variation, the existence of a 'standard' form of SG remains problematic.

Table 2.2 sets out different approaches to the issue of distinguishing between preference elicitation procedures. If utility measurement were an absolute requirement, and SG the recognized 'gold-standard'

Table 2.2 Hierarchy of preference elicitation procedures

	A SG as 'standard'	B Choice-based methods	C Preference elicitation
Standard gamble	1	1	1
Time trade-off	2	1	1
Category rating	3	2	1
Visual analogue scale	3	2	1
Conjoint methods	2a	1	1
Paired comparisons	3	1	1
Magnitude estimation	3	1	1
Equivalence matching	3	1	1

method, then all other procedures would generate approximations to (von Neumann-Morgenstern) utility (Column A). If a choice-based method were acceptable (Column B), then category rating and visual analogue scales would be relegated to the second tier. But if we are simply interested in capturing preference-based weights, and since this information can at least be inferred from any of the other methods, then there appears to be no way of distinguishing between these alternatives (Column C).

Thus, if utilities are an essential requirement for QALY computation, then there is no scope for admitting quality-adjustment weights based on methods other than the top ranked ones in (A). If social preferences are more widely interpreted, and methods that do not yield utilities are accepted as quality-adjustment weights, then (B) or (C) provide options.

'DEAD' AND HEALTH STATES WORSE THAN DEAD

The earliest conceptual models of health describe a continuum bounded by full health and dead.[4] By assigning values of 1 and 0 to these boundary states we define the unit interval in health state valuation. Empirical evidence of health states worse than dead emerged in the late 1970s, having been previously rejected as 'counter-intuitive'. Such states have negative values on a 0–1 metric. Dead or, more specifically, the value for dead, plays an important role in the measurement of values for health. First, it provides a descriptive anchor state that is present in some, but not all, health status classification systems. The simplest of these systems comprises two states – alive and dead. Dead is an essential descriptive component in any measure of health outcome. Health status measures that omit the state impose an artificial limit to the measurement of outcomes. More significantly, dead plays an important role in the derivation of values for non-fatal health states. This occurs either directly through the value elicitation methods used or indirectly through the process of data refinement and analysis used with the data such methods generate. The value for dead is pre-assigned to zero in TTO and in some forms of SG. Such methods allow no scope for non-zero values for dead, since they are designed around the concept of a 0–1 metric. Evidence from other preference elicitation methods, such as paired comparisons or visual analogue scaling, reveals that dead is not always the lowest ranked state and that it can take a non-zero value in those circumstances. The fact that, given the opportunity to do so, individuals record non-zero values for dead is, of course, troubling when set against the zero value imposed by TTO. However, this issue is effectively dealt with by introducing the assumption of equality of value of the distance between full health and dead. That assumption cannot be directly tested within TTO, but evidence from other valuation methods indicates some grounds for concern (Macran and Kind 2001). Eliciting values for dead is problematic in other methods too. Many studies reported by the EuroQoL Group[5] have noted the apparent reluctance of respondents to report a value for dead, even when using relatively undemanding rating scales. This selective non-response proves awkward to handle since the conversion of non-utility weights to a conventional 0–1 scale requires the presence of observed values for both boundary states. If an individual's value for full health or dead is missing, then their raw scores cannot be converted into a 0–1 equivalent. Hence, the conversion of preference data elicited by non-utility methods can introduce significant attrition if analysis is based on individual level data. A missing value for dead means the rejection of all values for non-fatal states recorded by that individual.

Valuation studies that identify health states worse than dead generate other difficulties relating to the interpretation of negative health state values. While positive health benefit can result from upward movement between health states with such values, movement between one such state and dead invites similar interpretation. It is this construction that fuels concerns about social preference data of this type and the suggestion that health economists are 'playing God'. This divergence has been circumvented by setting the value of all health states worse than dead to zero and, hence, negating the stated preferences for those states.

INTRA-METHOD DIFFERENCES

The set of methods used to elicit values for health can be broadly divided into two major groupings based on the claimed status of the resulting value set. Methods such as TTO and SG are widely held to generate utilities. The majority of other methods are regarded, at least by health economists, as generating a different (and by implication) lower order measurement of value. There are issues of comparison with, and between, these groups. The divergence of results obtained from TTO and SG procedures is well known. If both methods were applied to the valuation of a common set of health states, the ranking of resulting 'utilities' would probably be consistent between the two sets. However, the 'utilities' for mild health states are likely to be high in value (i.e. close to 1) given natural risk aversion and a reluctance to sacrifice life expectancy for what are regarded as relatively trivial health gains. TTO utilities are likely, too, to be lower than those resulting from SG. Such results could, of course, be portrayed as the manifestation of imperfect attempts to implement a standard procedure designed to elicit utility weights. Our understanding of the measurement error associated with one of these two methods for eliciting utilities requires that one is designated as the standard. However, there seems little evidence of a desire to reach such a conclusion. The measurement of utility weights is dominated by two distinct systems with separate units of measure. It is the ability to convert observations based on one system into corresponding values in the second that frees the user to select their favoured system. The failure of convergence between TTO and SG utilities ought to be disturbing for all users. The fact that it is apparently not so is of further concern. A conversion algorithm for utility weights generated by different procedures would seem to be an essential future requirement.

The second major group of valuation methods are not designed as mechanisms for generating utilities but even so are not free of the difficulties associated with claiming results in terms of a standard metric. Methods as different in practical terms as paired comparisons and magnitude estimation yield different estimates of value. An understanding of the relationship between values resulting from different methods is of interest but is by no means as critical as is the case with the measurement of utility. Here convergence is a windfall gain. Failure of convergence is neither inconvenient nor damning. Different valuation methods simply can, and do, yield different results. In point of fact, early studies of valuation sought to explain the relationship between the results obtained from different valuation methods (Blischke *et al.* 1975). In part, such studies drew on the experience of experiments in psychophysics that tested subjective responses to physical stimuli such as pain, light and sound (Stevens 1966). The suggestion that a single power function governs the transformation of subjective judgements across preference modalities was always going to be far-fetched, although there is some supportive evidence from cross-modality matching experiments. The use of category rating as an indirect method of generating utility weights draws it authority from psychophysics, resting as it does on a power function transformation to convert values into utilities. The existence of a single transformation function would, of course, prove to be highly convenient, but there is conflicting evidence concerning both the form of such a function and, in the case of a power function, the value of the exponent. The use of category rating as an alternate to measuring utility is far from proven and its credibility relies heavily on past custom and practice.

At the root of much of the difficulty in resolving differences in valuations for health that emerge from these two classes of measurement procedure is a failure to establish the defining properties of utility measurement. When confronted with a set of weights described as being utilities, what test can be applied to establish the veracity of the claim? How do we know if these are utilities or not? The suggestion appears to be that the measurement characteristics of a given set of weights flow from the nature of the procedure used to establish them. Hence, procedures that generate utilities necessarily yield utilities. There is no external test of the utility measurement property. A utility is a utility is a utility. The interpretation of utility weights as having universal standard value has not yet been established and all the evidence points to this being a difficult case to make.

SOURCE(S) OF PREFERENCE VALUES

In the specific setting of NICE appraisals there can be little room for doubt or manoeuvre. The source of social preferences is clearly the general public. This leaves little scope for other options that have been used to determine quality-adjustment weights for the purposes of QALY calculations. The use of patients or other (indirect) beneficiaries of treatment as a source of such weights clearly violates the NICE requirement. Apart from this obvious inconsistency there is the question of response shift and other systematic biases that are likely to influence the value of the quality-adjustments. Such is the strength of the imperative to obtain a number (any number) that consideration of these issues is seldom, if ever, made in reviewing the status of quality of life data in appraisal documentation. If patients were a non-admissible source of quality-adjustment weights then so, too, would be the expert panel.

The notion of using the general population as the required source for social preferences is intuitively appealing but somewhat problematic. It is not clear how such an exercise should be conducted.

Sampling non-institutionalized members of the community leads to the exclusion of potential 'voters' who are in prison, in hospital or other long-stay health facilities, in residential homes or in the armed services. Such groups are often excluded in other population surveys that are described as being 'national' in character. More difficult for the instrument developer, and for the end-user who seeks to conform to the NICE requirement, is the extent to which the *achieved sample* can be regarded as representative of society as a whole. This *ex post* assessment is especially critical where preference elicitation methods, or other aspects of survey design, lead to a high rate of attrition in the acquired data.

The fact that social preferences have been collected from a large, representative sample of the general population does not mean that those values are fixed for all time. There is continuous movement around the subject of health, illness, longevity and death in terms of public debate and comment. This suggests that, while the rank order of health states may remain reassuringly stable, the distances between health states and, hence, their relative values can be expected to change over time. So, the age of social preferences may be just as important as their source.

Although NICE requires the social preferences to be those of the relevant population, is it safe to accept population values imported from beyond the boundaries of England and Wales? It is tempting to propose a hierarchical response to this question in which, say, the populations of Canada, New Zealand or Holland might be favoured over those of Japan, Hungary or Slovenia. However, given their distinct national identities, it is difficult to envisage how a case could be made for any other than a local, domestic UK population being used as the source of preference values.

The portability of social preferences across national boundaries has been the subject of investigation (Brooks *et al.* 2003), and there is evidence that suggests that health states attract similar values in different European countries. Where preferences have been generated in national population surveys conducted outside the UK (or, more restrictively, England and Wales), it would be necessary to demonstrate that the achieved sample at least broadly shared the same personal and environmental characteristics as the UK. An Australian population study might yield values that were acceptable for domestic applications, but external evidence of convergence with the UK would be needed before ascribing any legitimacy to the use of those values in NICE appraisals. The absence of evidence to show that the *source* of preference values can be safely treated as approximating the general population of England and Wales ought to act as a filter that automatically degrades the status of those preference values.

The source of reference weights promulgated for these measures is equally varied. The valuation of EQ-5D health states has been the subject of UK population surveys. Although the definitive 1993 MVH survey (Williams 1997) embraces a subset of values from Scotland it probably represents the approach to the derivation of social values for EQ-5D health states that most closely matches the requirements for NICE appraisals (NICE 2004). Other measures, such as HUI, that are based on utility elicitation have yet to be calibrated in terms of UK population preferences.

AGGREGATION

If capturing individual preferences for health states is accepted as technically feasible, the issue regarding how best to represent the collective preferences of a group remains open. The choice of measure of central tendency is often portrayed as a consequential to the distributional form of the data and/or the nature of the underlying measurement that it represents. The choice of aggregate measure is widest where data lies on a cardinal scale and, for normally distributed data of this type, the mean and median will be very similar. Where the distribution is skewed, then some appropriate remedial transformation might be applied to compensate for it. However, this type of post-processing may modify the structure of the data – a state of affairs that would be vigorously challenged were these data to be regarded as analogous to the preferences recorded in government elections. Extremes of political opinion, as with values for health, are likely to be encountered. While their acceptability to the majority may be in doubt, the legitimacy of individuals who hold those views cannot be questioned. Some individuals hold views that lead them to express values of health that differ dramatically from others. For example, the values of psychiatric nurses were sometimes several orders of magnitude higher than those of medical nurses (Rosser and Kind 1978). Since neither can be compared to a standard set of values, we accept that they are a reflection of the diversity that occurs naturally across society. 'Correcting' for that diversity would be to compromise the very rationale that motivates the collection of values for health. The use of the pooled mean in this case would give disproportionate importance to the values of one set of nurses over the other. The median would be a fairer method of representing the collective view across nurses, allowing extremes to count but also treating all 'voters' on an equal footing.

STABILITY OF PREFERENCES

If it is to be expected that different methods of eliciting values for health yield different numeric estimates, does this represent the limit of any concern with the stability of preference data? Little is known about the stability of preferences in respect of other factors. Investigation of the stability of utilities in patients over relatively short-term time horizons has been conducted (Llewellyn-Thomas *et al.* 1993), but it remains unclear whether or not social preferences are modified over time and, if so, the magnitude of the time interval over which such changes operate. Evidence at York from visual analogue scale ratings data in population studies indicates little change in aggregate values over a five-year period. The evidence from TTO is less compelling. It is important to establish the extent of any temporally induced shift in social preference weights. The determination of current priorities might, otherwise, be inappropriately informed by values representing the preferences of society in earlier time periods. At the very least we should be able to indicate the likely size of any shift in social preferences. As with the presentation of data on costing, and, as a future safeguard in the interpretation of analysis based on any social values, the year(s) to which those values relate should be clearly reported.

The same good practice could be extended in identifying the national context for those social preference weights. In the case of EQ-5D, for example, for some countries there are no domestic estimates of the values for the health states that it defines. In the absence of any more appropriate set of values, those generated as part of the MVH study in the UK have become a default option. Where that option is exercised it is incumbent on users to make that choice explicit and to address any relevant issues that are linked to it. For example, the use of utility weights from one European country might be somewhat questionable in other countries with different social and cultural norms. Further, as the UK weights age, it might be that other, more recent, social preference weights represent a better default.

Within national population studies it will be important to establish the extent of any systematic differences in social preference weights for health. This issue may be partly resolved if weights are aggregated at the national level and are based on data collected from a representative population sample. However, with increased emphasis on devolution, the capacity to compare local or regional values with those of a national preference set will become more important. There are other population subgroups to consider. Health variations associated with social class, education, housing and income can impact on values assigned to health. While the emphasis on social preferences indicates a whole population approach, it is important to track any systematic differences that might emerge from the application of alternative preferences sets that reflect the views of key subgroups.

ACCURACY OF PREFERENCE VALUES

The concept of accuracy in the measurement of health status is itself difficult, given the absence of single standard definition. However, beyond the description of health, the notion of accuracy in respect of the valuation is problematic. The detection of error depends upon calibration with respect to some reference measurement, which is absent in the valuation of health. At the level of the individual taking part in a health valuation study, it is important to consider the scope for variability in their responses. A variety of factors will influence their performance in executing any valuation task. The method itself may induce uncertainty through a failure in understanding of its mechanics. The concept of health valuation lies outside the everyday experience of most individuals and the description of health used in any study may provoke unintended and unobservable consequences for those taking part. Attempts to establish the robustness of estimates of value rely on their reproducibility on a second occasion. Test-retest exposure is a requirement in virtually all studies of valuation and this testing provides reassurance when the two sets of values are broadly in line. However, the process of engaging in a health valuation exercise may lead to a shift in attitude towards health, with a resulting difference between test-retest results. Similarly, much concern is directed towards the consistency of individual responses. By implication, inconsistent responses indicate inaccurate estimates of value. Apparent violations of logical consistency may be taken as evidence bearing on the valuation protocol itself as much as on the performance of those taking part in it.

The notion of accuracy also operates at the level of the health status measurement system. Generic systems such as HUI, EQ-5D, and SF-6D are based on descriptive classifications that vary in content and scale. Claims for greater accuracy tend to be associated with systems that embody larger sets of health states. It is tempting to consider that more dimensions, and more levels within dimensions, lead to greater accuracy in classifying health status, but this can prove to be illusionary. If the differential value between two states cannot be established in a meaningful way, then increasing their descriptive complexity may not improve the 'accuracy' of its use. Taking the 0–1 metric as the typical space in which health state values are located, this allows for 100 unique values represented to two places of decimal. It seems unlikely that our capacity to discriminate value differences matches even this level of 'accuracy'. More probable is that values within a certain range would be regarded as virtually synonymous if re-presented to participants in a valuation study. Are two health states with a value difference of (say) 0.05 perceived as different? Is the dominance relationship inferred by their values recognized? The issue then is less about the accuracy of the estimates of social preference weights and more about the extent to which those weights are capable of representing changes in health status.

A GENERIC REFERENCE CASE TECHNOLOGY

Finally, there is the issue of how best to bring order to the potentially chaotic use of health values data in practice. Recent guidance offered by NICE (2004) proposes a reference case approach, as foreshadowed by the earlier Washington Panel. It is difficult, in principle, to argue against such a development, since it offers the prospect that all appraisals will be based on a shared, common method of measuring health outcomes. However, it is the definition of that common method that invokes a degree of concern about the appraisal process. If the unit of account is defined in terms of utility then it logically follows that the process by which utility weights are elicited is of importance. Here the choice is not simply whether TTO or SG weights constitute the standard, it is the specification of the procedure by which those weights are derived. This would require a step-change in standardizing the measurement of utility that would, in effect, foreclose on some of the issues that so far remain indeterminate. The evidence for such a courageous stand is simply not available. Hence, for the time being, it appears that TTO and SG utilities will be given equal status. It would be troubling were this parity to extend to estimates of utility derived from other valuation methods, such as category rating, unless the scientific case can be established.

If the reference case approach does not involve the advocacy of one standard system of measurement, then there should be a degree of standardization by taking a less inflexible line. With respect to the measurement of utility, rather than direct attention to a single set of weights, it might be argued that control can be exercised by attending to the procedures by which utilities are estimated. In this situation the reference case approach would require that utilities are estimated in accordance with a particular methodology. This would be a potentially more difficult system to police but one in which some degree of flexibility was retained for those applications in which a prescribed set of utility weights was problematic. Logically, too, a procedure-based standardization would have to extend to the descriptive classification that formed the basis of the measurement system.

The need for a standardized approach to the measurement of health status in an economic evaluation system has long been evident. The seeming luxury of a 1000 cost/QALY estimates (Tengs and Wallace 2000) simply emphasizes the restricted capacity to make comparisons across evidence generated in different locations, using different methodologies. The reference case approach at least encourages the use of standard measures – not to the exclusion of other measures, but as a preliminary, required task. Movement away from the reference case will need to be justified and many of the issues touched upon in this chapter provide the basis for such a justification. The substantive research agenda remains intact.

CONCLUSIONS

The situation that we face as practitioners and researchers in the field of health economics can be portrayed in two mutually exclusive ways. Social preferences needed for the computation of QALYs must be expressed in terms of utilities derived from a choice-based methodology linked to relevant theory. In this situation, it would be likely that the method by which utilities are generated would follow as a logical progression from theory into practice. This fortunate state of affairs would be further complemented by a high degree of consensus in academic circles about the theoretical basis of such measurement and practical ways of achieving it. Furthermore, novel techniques could be empirically tested against existing standards as a mechanism for determining their suitability as substitutes. The alternative position admits that social preferences *may* be expressed as utilities but that this is not an *absolute* requirement. The value associated with a health state may be determined by a larger set of methods, the only constraint being that it must produce a single index value on a scale that assigns a value of 0 and 1 to dead and full health respectively. Both alternatives leave us well short of an agreed or sustainable position. Since procedures for preference measurement tend to generate different values for a given health state, it will require an extraordinary piece of good fortune to come up with a plausible explanation, or a unifying theory, that allows for transformation between competing value sets. It could be that a retreat into an exclusive utility-based approach has some merit, since this would reduce the range of candidate methods. However, it would still leave us some way short of an accepted (or acceptable) common method.

In the absence of a recognized standard, then multiple measurement methods are tolerated as having some claim to legitimacy. The occasional happy accidental convergence of results offers some comfort that perhaps the picture is less complicated than others would have us believe. Widely differing results give further support for the view that different methods necessarily yield divergent results. The usual response to such a multiplicity of choice is to take refuge in sensitivity analysis rather than to attack the problem head on. Does it make any difference to the conclusions if we apply one set of values/utilities or another? Accepting the luxury of this approach leads to the inescapable conclusion that the choice of preference elicitation method is an irrelevancy and that, ultimately, any number will do.

All this may be dismissed as navel-gazing at best and, at worst, an assault on the foundations of health outcome measurement. The valuation of health is often portrayed as a rather weak form of measurement, subjective and malleable in character. It is contrasted with more substantive, reliable forms of measurement conducted by traditional scientific methods. The certainty of expressing measurement in terms of well-calibrated physical units is preferred to the measurement of values for health and, by extension, the measurement of health status or HRQL. Such a posture belies the evidence. For example, the measurement of blood pressure can be made through a multiplicity of different methods. It is characterized by well-documented errors in administration, and in the recording of observations. It is subject to variability associated with the time of day, the handedness and weight of the patient, their posture and by the appearance of the individual measuring the blood pressure.[6] All this is despite a *de facto* gold-standard taught to medical personnel the world over. Set against the high aspirations and achievements in the investigation of the value of health, any claim for a 'harder' scientific status in clinical practice is difficult to sustain.

The relevance for health economists of the issues rehearsed here will be determined by context and by application. From the vantage point of the theorist, the seeming uncertainty acts to emphasize the richness of the field. For the decision-maker, these issues may appear to be trifling distractions, diverting attention away from other (and by implication) more fundamental problems. Why worry too much about questions concerning the value of health outcomes in poorly conducted clinical studies? After all, the impact of variable data quality can be studied through sensitivity analysis, and imperfections in the outcomes data can be addressed through this mechanism. This response deals with the short-run implications but leaves the issues unresolved. To raise awareness of these problems is not to take away from the immenseness of the achievements of the past 30 years – rather, it is a constructive remedy against complacency.

DISCUSSION
Martin Buxton

The progress made and the outstanding issues in the field of health state valuation represent important topics for a stock-taking exercise in this volume of chapters celebrating the CHE anniversary, not least because of the major contribution that York economists have made over the years to this work. In particular, Alan Williams, with a succession of co-researchers, not least Paul Kind, has pushed forward the thinking from early conceptualization (Culyer *et al.* 1972), through the opportunistic use of a 'convenience' instrument ('the Rosser Matrix') (Kind *et al.* 1982), through the establishment of and active participation in the Euro-Qol Group and the development of the EQ-5D, to the landmark Measurement and Valuation of Health Project to establish UK population representative values for EQ-5D health states (Williams 1997). This chapter is therefore very welcome.

The questions it raises are important, though they constitute a revisiting of well-trodden ground. Nevertheless, one can't but help feeling that this is a case of researchers wanting to have their cake and eat it. For years, health economists have argued that QALYs should be used as a measure of the effect of health interventions and that allocation decisions should be based on incremental cost per QALY. Now that decision-makers have been persuaded of the value of these approaches, there is an anguished wringing of hands fearing that these decision-makers, while astute enough to adopt the methodology, may not be astute enough to use it wisely. Users may not adequately appreciate that the QALY is a fragile species, whose precise manifestation may be a temporary phenomenon depending upon the underlying descriptive systems, the methods used to elicit values and the group from whom those values are elicited.

Of course there is a danger that decision-makers may be naïve or simply choose to ignore real complications. Taking the use of health state valuations in the technology appraisal work of NICE as the key UK context, which seems to have been one of the spurs to the chapter, we need to ask whether a concern about the way this evidence is used is justified.

Certainly, NICE has not taken away the economists' ball and left them out of the game. On the contrary, it is a body that has drawn so many economists into its non-executive board, to its secretariat, to its standing appraisal and guideline committees, not counting those employed in providing evidence on behalf of the stakeholders or assessment teams, that a real concern has been that it is distorting the balance of health economics away from other important areas of research (Appleby and Devlin 2004). Nor am I aware of any specific cases where it appears that NICE has over-simplistically relied on the accuracy of specific utility estimates, although it would be a useful task to review a series of NICE appraisals and check how sensitive the decisions might have been to the usually unstated uncertainty surrounding key utility values.

Rather, what we observe is a decision-making body embracing the 'cost per QALY' methodology (and with it using the underlying research on health state valuations) to address its task. Thoroughly advised by a range of economists, NICE has clarified its own extra-welfarist viewpoint and embodied it in guidance, which now reinforces NICE's position with the clear definition of a 'reference case' to maximize comparability (NICE 2004). We can all quibble and argue about details of NICE's precise position, but it has adopted a wholly informed and rational strategy.

In these circumstances, what is now incumbent upon the research community if they wish to see NICE's strategy work and the use of cost per QALY estimates evolve appropriately, is to work with NICE, not harking back to long-standing arguments and worries, but identifying the key issues that affect, and might undermine, their decisions as they use the available research evidence. It may not be a perfect tool but, after some 30 years or so of research investment, it does now offer some practical assistance to those making very difficult but necessary recommendations about the adoption of new technologies.

So, as we contemplate an imperfect but useful tool, being used to make serious decisions in the National Health Service (NHS), the question we should be asking is not whether the tool is perfect, but rather whether it is better than the alternative. NICE's embrace of QALYs, warts and all, seems to me to be a case where the imperfections of the tool are minor when compared with the way such decisions have been made in the past. So yes, we do need to continue research to improve our armoury of health state classification systems and health state value elicitation instruments, to provide robust algorithms that translate and recalibrate values between instruments, to continue to build up and maintain a database of current values for populations and specific subgroups within them, and to better represent the uncertainty around these values. But in our striving to improve matters we should be wary of appearing to baulk when users intelligently apply the current state of the art: rather we should applaud them. And if, on occasions, we observe decision-makers forgetting the caveats and the uncertainties, the onus is on the many economists, within and around the NICE enterprise, to alert them to those particular situations where the remaining weaknesses in the tool may impact on the decisions being made.

NOTES

1 This text was revised taking into account the comments of Professor Martin Buxton, Brunel University, who acted as the discussant for the original paper presented at the CHE conference. I am also grateful for comments from Professor John Brazier, University of Sheffield.

2 The term 'tariff' has such demonstrably negative associations that its continued usage needs to be denied. A less objectionable term might be 'social preference weights'.
3 For example, TTO procedures at McMaster differ from those used at York.
4 There is an important distinction between death and dead. The former is an event, whereas the latter is a state.
5 Established in 1987, the EuroQol Group comprises a network of international, multi-lingual, multi-disciplinary researchers, committed to the development and application of the EQ-5D.
6 The phenomenon of 'white-coated' hypertension is well documented.

REFERENCES

Appleby, J. and Devlin, N. (2004) British health economists: is what they do what they should be doing? CES-HESG Meeting, Paris.

Blischke, W.R., Bush, J.W. and Kaplan, R.M. (1975) A successive intervals analysis of social preference measures for a health status index, *Health Services Research*, 10(2): 181–98.

Brazier, J., Roberts, J. and Deverill, M. (2002) The estimation of a preference-based measure of health from the SF-36, *Journal of Health Economics*, 21(2): 271–92.

Brooks, R. (1996) EuroQol: the current state of play, *Health Policy*, 37(1), 53–72.

Brooks, R., Rabin, R. and de Charro, F. (2003) *The Measurement and Valuation of Health Status Using EQ-5D: A European Perspective*. Dordrecht: Kluwer.

Culyer, A.J., Lavers, R. and Williams, A.H. (1972) Social indicators: health, *Social Trends*, 2: 31–42.

Dolan, P., Gudex, C., Kind, P. and Williams, A.H. (1996) Valuing health states: a comparison of methods, *Journal of Health Economics*, 15: 209–31.

Fanshel, S. and Bush, J. (1970) A health status index and its application to health services outcomes, *Operations Research*, 18: 1021.

Gold, M.R., Russell, L.B. and Weinstein, M.C. (1996) *Cost-effectiveness in Health and Medicine*. New York: Oxford University Press.

Green, P., Carmone, F.J. and Smith, S.M. ([1970] 1989) *Multi-dimensional Scaling: Concepts and Applications*. Boston, MA: Allyn & Bacon.

Grogono, A.W. and Woodgate, D.J. (1971) Index for measuring health, *Lancet*, 2: 1024.

Hadorn, D.C., Hays, R.D., Uebersax, J. and Hauber, T. (1992) Improving task comprehension in the measurement of health state preferences. A trial of informational cartoon figures and a paired-comparison task. *Journal of Clinical Epidemiology*, 45(3): 233–43.

Kind, P., Rosser, R. and Williams, A. (1982) Valuation of quality of life:

some psychometric evidence, in M. Jones-Lee (ed.) *The Value of Life & Safety*, pp. 159–70. Holland: North-Holland Publishing Company.

Llewellyn-Thomas, H.A., Sutherland, H.J. and Thiel, E.C. (1993) Do patients' evaluations of a future health state change when they actually enter that state? *Medical Care*, 31(11): 1002–12.

Macran, S. and Kind, P. (2001) 'Death' and the valuation of health-related quality of life, *Medical Care*, 39(3): 217–22.

McKenna, S.P., Hunt, S.M. and McEwen, J. (1981) Weighting the serious-ness of perceived health problems using Thurstone's method of paired comparisons, *International Journal of Epidemiology*, 10(1): 93–7.

NICE (National Institute for Clinical Excellence) (2004) *Guide to the Methods of Technology Appraisal*. London: NICE.

Rosser, R.M. and Kind, P. (1978) A scale of valuations of states of illness: is there a social consensus? *International Journal of Epidemiology*, 7: 347–58.

Rosser, R.M. and Watts, V.C. (1972) The measurement of hospital output, *International Journal of Epidemiology*, 1(4): 361–8.

Stevens, S.S. (1966) A metric for the social consensus, *Science*, 151: 530–41.

Tengs, T. and Wallace, A. (2000) One thousand health-related quality-of-life estimates, *Medical Care*, 38(6): 583–637.

Thurstone, L.L. (1927) Method of paired comparisons for social values, *Journal of Abnormal Social Psychology*, 21: 384–400.

Torrance, G.W., Sackett, D.L. and Thomas, W.H. (1973) Utility maximiza-tion model for program evaluation: a demonstration application, in *Health Status Indexes*, pp. 156–65. Chicago: Hospital Research and Education Trust.

von Neumann, J. and Morgenstern, O. (1944) *Theory of Games and Economic Behavior*. Princeton, NJ: Princeton University Press.

Williams, A.H. (1997) *The Measurement and Valuation of Health: A Chronicle*. Centre for Health Economics Discussion Paper 136. York: Centre for Health Economics (CHE).

3

ELICITING EQUITY-EFFICIENCY TRADE-OFFS IN HEALTH

Alan Williams, Aki Tsuchiya and Paul Dolan[1]

INTRODUCTION

Health systems typically pursue two broad objectives: to maximize
the health of the population served, and to reduce inequalities in
health within that population. It is virtually certain that there is
conflict between achievement of these two objectives, so that – in
setting policy – an explicit weight should be given to each. Our particular interest in this chapter is, therefore, what weight policymakers
seeking to allocate health system resources should give to health
maximization relative to the reduction of health inequalities. We first
discuss the policy problem, and then the underlying philosophical
principles. Some economic theory is adduced to illustrate the principles, and some empirical analysis based on that theory is then presented. We conclude with a discussion of the implications for policy.

THE POLICY PROBLEM

As Chapter 2 explained, cost-effectiveness analysis (CEA) is moving
centre-stage in many countries, as policymakers seek to allocate their
limited resources to maximum effect. However, traditional cost-
effectiveness analysis (CEA) considers only the maximization of
health gains, and treats such gains equally, whoever receives them. In
contrast, in many countries, there is great policy preoccupation with

health inequalities as well as health improvement. The question is: how can these equity considerations be integrated into traditional cost-effectiveness methods?

In England and Wales, the National Institute for Clinical Excellence (NICE) assists policymakers by making judgements on the clinical and cost-effectiveness of the interventions referred to it by government ministers (see www.nice.org.uk). It has developed a rough rule of thumb that an intervention is deemed to be cost-effective if it can produce additional quality-adjusted life years (QALYs) for less than £20k each, although in certain cases it is willing to go up to £30k (NICE 2003). The case law from past decisions has not yet generated any very clear guidance as to what the exceptional circumstances are that might justify such a 'bonus', or by how much.

One possible justification for such a loosening of its threshold value for a QALY might be a consideration of 'equity', which NICE is also charged with taking into account in its decisions. This is certainly not part of the standard cost per QALY calculations that emerge from the data presented to it as part of its appraisal process. Indeed, the standard practice is to treat all QALYs as equal in value no matter who receives them. There is, however, no reason in principle why that needs be the end of the story.

In practice, NICE will not get much help concerning equity from a typical economic evaluation of a health care intervention, since economic evaluations focus exclusively on health maximization. The justifications for this neglect of equity are many and varied. The most fundamental is a denial that economics has any tools to handle such issues, since its current mainstream corpus of knowledge derives from a position in which interpersonal comparisons of welfare are held to be invalid and so are ruled out of consideration. But those willing and able to emancipate themselves from this strict welfarist regime still face severe problems in addressing issues of equity, because equity is an essentially contestable concept in which many rival views flourish. In the present context we simplify matters somewhat by concentrating attention on ethical issues which focus on outcomes rather than procedures.

In this context there are two broad streams of philosophical thought that appear to be relevant: that concerned with 'desert' and that concerned with 'egalitarianism'. NICE has already taken a position on one manifestation of 'desert', by determining that people should not be discriminated against on the grounds that their medical condition is 'self-induced' (e.g. smoking-related diseases) (NICE 2002). Whether it is ethical for an appraisal to take into account the extent to which (say) continued smoking affects the efficacy of the treatment, which is an issue that should be addressed in any calculation of cost-effectiveness, is a question still left open. There may be other manifestations of 'desert' (which NICE may wish to consider), concerned for instance with 'rule of rescue' considerations and which we discuss in the next section.

The dominant policy issue in the egalitarian realm, however, is undoubtedly the reduction in inequalities in health, usually measured by differences in life expectancy at birth and most often focused on differences between the social classes (DHSS 1980; Independent Inquiry into Inequalities in Health 1998). Focusing on inequalities in outcome is more fundamental than focusing on inequalities in access, or resources, or utilization, which are best seen as instrumental. Indeed, it may be necessary to make the distribution of these 'instruments' *more unequal* in order to reduce inequalities in the fundamental variable, which is a person's lifetime experience of health.

PHILOSOPHICAL PRINCIPLES

The philosophical position that is particularly useful as the framework within which to discuss ethical issues concerning inequalities in people's lifetime experience of health is the 'fair innings argument' (FIA)(Glover 1977; Harris 1985). Broadly speaking, it asserts that everyone is entitled to a certain span of life (say 70 years) and anyone dying before that age has died 'prematurely' and should be considered not to have had 'a fair innings' from life. Conversely, those living to a ripe old age have had more than 'a fair innings' and when they die cannot be said to have been treated unfairly. So, the appropriate unit of analysis should be a person's whole lifetime experience of health, rather than how they happen to be at the moment. The version of the FIA to which we subscribe is not based simply on lifetime measured in years, however, but upon *quality-adjusted* lifetime measured in QALYs (Williams 1997; Tsuchiya 2000). Someone who has spent 70 years wracked by pain and severely disabled cannot be said to have been treated by life as fairly as someone whose 70 years have been relatively free of such suffering.

A person's lifetime experience of health is made up of two elements: their actual accumulated experience to date (preferably measured in QALYs) and their expected future health (also measured in QALYs) given their history and their current health status. The sum of these two is a person's expected lifetime experience of health at current age (measured in QALYs).

Reducing inequalities in people's lifetime experience of health means that we have to discriminate in *favour* of those with poor prospects and *against* those with good prospects. On average, people's likelihood of achieving a 'fair innings' improves with age, and some people will already have achieved it. The latter will all be older members of society, so the FIA calls for discrimination against them and in favour of younger people with poorer prospects, all on the grounds of distributive justice, in this case focused on intergenerational equity.

But it may be that, from the standpoint of public policy, some inequalities in lifetime experience of health may be regarded as more inequitable than others, either because of their size or because of their nature. Small differences, which are largely the fault of disadvantaged people, may not be regarded as equally important issues for public policy as large differences caused by factors over which individuals have no control. This would mean that the 'fair innings' norm might be different for different groups of people, and one interesting issue is whether the norm should be the same for men and women (Tsuchiya and Williams 2004). These are matters that public policy has to address, and which, in a democratic society, require informed dialogue.

A more problematic notion is the so-called 'rule of rescue', which asserts that, in order to demonstrate that we are a caring community, there are occasions when it is necessary to commit resources generously to rescue someone in dire peril, *without* counting the costs too closely (McKie and Richardson 2003). It is debatable whether this is an argument that should apply to a body like NICE, which is explicitly charged with making careful evidence-based calculations of costs and benefits for decision-making at the national level. What might be regarded as a humane and generous gesture at an individual level may be regarded as a capricious and irresponsible act for a deliberative body advising on how best to spend taxpayers' money. Against this it might be argued that we should *deliberately and systematically* attempt to 'rescue', say, the prematurely terminally ill. However, it must always be remembered that according preferential status to groups whose health gains are small in relation to their costs means depriving others of much larger health gains. This is because, by implication, it is saying that the latter are less deserving people, and the consequent reduction in the health status of the population as a whole is a sacrifice worth making. It requires a moral case to be established as to why this should be so.

ECONOMIC THEORY

The social welfare function (SWF) is a conceptual tool in welfare economics that can be used to represent the competing objectives of health maximization and reduction of inequalities simultaneously. It therefore helps us to set up a policy model that will serve as the theoretical basis for empirical work to estimate the implied trade-offs.

It is conventional in microeconomic theory to represent the welfare of an individual or of a group by drawing a 'map' in which the contours indicate different levels of social welfare. Figure 3.1 is such a map, in which social welfare depends on the health of two (groups of) people, A and B, with their respective levels of health plotted on the axes. Each point in the map represents a particular combination of the health of A and the health of B. The contours (W_1, W_2 and W_3) each plot out the locus of points which are combinations of A's health and B's health that society regard as equally desirable (or in other words between which they are indifferent). Since better health means higher welfare, contours further away from the origin represent higher social welfare.

In Figure 3.1, these social welfare contours have a rather special property, in that they are symmetrical about a 45° line from the origin. Along this 45° line, the health of A and the health of B are identical. Having the contours curve as they do in this diagram means that if this society had a given amount of health to share between A and B, they would prefer it to be divided equally. To test this, consider a situation where a fixed amount of health is available,

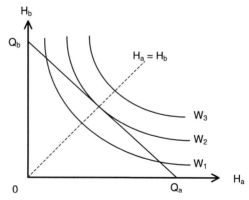

Figure 3.1   Social welfare contours

and that Q_a and Q_b each represent the case where all health went to A or to B. The straight line joining Q_a to Q_b represents all the ways in which this total can be divided between A and B. Along this line the highest contour is reached when $H_a = H_b$ (contour W_2).

Suppose that the present situation, depicted by the point S in Figure 3.2, is that the health of A is much worse than the health of B, and that this situation lies on the contour W_2. At the point S that contour has a slope indicated by the straight line drawn as a tangent to the contour at that point. Its slope represents the rate at which the health of A and the health of B can be substituted for each other and still leave us on the same contour, if we are at the point S. If its slope is −2, this means that we would be prepared to sacrifice two units of B's health in order to improve A's health by one unit. If we implemented a policy which moved us along W_2 and closer to the perfect equality line ($H_a = H_b$), then the slope of the W_2 contour at such a point would decline, and we would be less willing to sacrifice B's health to improve A's. In the extreme, when both are equal in health, the slope becomes −1 and we regard changes in either as of equal value. Thus, these contours represent a situation in which the greater is the inequality the greater is the rate at which we would sacrifice the health of the better off to improve the health of the worse off. It is this rate of trade-off that forms the basis for a set of 'equity weights' which indicate how much weight should be given to a health gain depending on the characteristics of the recipient. In the simple example shown here, the weight attached to a gain for A should be twice that of the weight given to a gain for B.

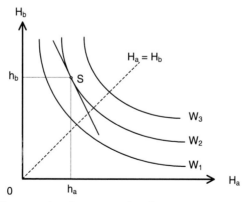

Figure 3.2 Representing the current situation

This very simple case can be generalized in a number of ways. Briefly, the more complex situations can be represented as follows: (a) increasing or decreasing a society's aversion to inequalities in health is represented by increasing or decreasing the curvature of the contours; (b) treating the health of one group as more important than that of the other by making the contours tilt to one side, so that they become asymmetrical with respect to the 45° line from the origin; and (c) if changing the distribution of health can only be achieved by sacrificing some health in aggregate, then the line $Q_a.Q_b$ of Figure 3.1 will no longer be straight but will have to be redrawn accordingly. The important thing here is that each of the properties of the diagram can be varied to fit the policy situation that is of interest, and empirical work can be focused on each of the important parameters.

WHAT THE PUBLIC THINK

With this analytical background in mind, our chosen task is to find out what the views of the public are regarding inequalities in lifetime health between different subgroups of the population. (For a more general review of the related literature, see Dolan *et al.* 2004.) A critical issue is whether they see all inequalities in health as equally inequitable, or whether some are regarded as more inequitable than others.

We began by investigating what notions of 'fairness' the general public thought should influence National Health Service (NHS) policy. In this early work, we sought to explore how respondents interpret questions that are put to them. This was done by giving them time to think about what was being asked of them and the opportunity to reflect upon their responses. To achieve this, ten focus groups with a total of 60 participants were convened (Cookson and Dolan 1999, 2000; Dolan *et al.* 1999). Each group met on two occasions with a fortnight between each meeting and three main issues were covered.

First, we administered the same questionnaire at the beginning of the first meeting and at the end of the second meeting in order to look at the effect of discussion and deliberation on people's views. We found that respondents became more reticent about the role that their views should play in determining priorities and more sympathetic towards the role that managers play. About half of the respondents initially wanted to give lower priority to smokers, heavy drinkers and illegal drug users, but after discussion many no longer wished to discriminate against such people. If the considered opinions of the general public are required, then doubt is cast on those surveys that do not allow respondents the time or opportunity to reflect upon their responses.

Second, the groups were asked to discuss a hypothetical rationing choice, concerning four identified patients. It was explained to respondents that the purpose of the exercise was to find out what general ethical principles they support. On the basis of an innovative qualitative data analysis, which translates what people say into ethical principles identified in the theoretical literature, the public appear to support three main rationing principles: (i) a broad 'rule of rescue' that gives priority to those in immediate need, (ii) health maximization and (iii) equalization of lifetime health.

Third, the groups were asked to consider priority setting across groups rather than individuals. Respondents were asked to imagine two groups of patients who would both benefit from treatment but by differing amounts. Respondents were told that only half of the patients could be treated and they were asked to decide whether they would choose to give the same priority to both groups or to give priority to the group that could gain the most from treatment. A clear message came through from the data – that equality of access should prevail over the maximization of benefits. However, this was subject to the outcome constraint that treatments are sufficiently effective.

Our major exploratory study, financed by the Economic and Social Research Council (ESRC), sought to examine the relative importance placed by the public on different forms of equity, and to consider the extent to which they are prepared to trade off efficiency (or health maximization) against equity in the distribution of health care resources (Shaw *et al.* 2001; Dolan *et al.* 2002; Dolan and Tsuchiya 2003). The main preference elicitation stages of the project involved face-to-face interviews with a representative sample of 130 York residents, and a postal questionnaire using very similar questions to the interviews, which was returned by a nationally representative sample of 833 people.

The main questions in the face-to-face interviews were concerned with eliciting the degree of inequality aversion, so that the parameters in an SWF could be determined. The questions presented information on differences in health between two groups to elicit the extent to which respondents are prepared to sacrifice overall health gain in order to reduce inequalities in health. The general structure of the interview was that each respondent was asked questions relating to: inequalities in life expectancy at birth by social class or by sex; inequalities in rates of long-term illness by social class or by smoking status; inequalities in rates of childhood mortality by social class; and the treatment of two groups of people, one that has taken care of their health and one that has not. The different variants meant that we could test whether the SWF has a different shape depending on how health is represented and how the groups are defined.

In the first three questions, respondents were asked to choose between two programmes that brought about the same overall health gain, but one benefited both groups equally while the other targeted the group with the worst health prospects. If the targeted programme was chosen, the benefit from this programme was successively reduced until the respondent chose the untargeted programme, or until all response options were exhausted. In the fourth question, respondents were told that there are two groups of people in equal health. The groups are the same in all relevant respects except that those in the first group (A) have not cared for their health, while those in the second group (B) have taken care of their health. Without an intervention, all individuals are expected to die soon, but there are not enough resources to save everyone. Respondents were asked to choose between two programmes: one that will save 100 lives from group A and one that will save q lives from group B. To identify the relative importance of these programmes, respondents were offered a series of pairwise choices between $p = 100$ and decreasing values of q.

The results suggest that there is a general willingness to sacrifice health benefits to target those with the worst health prospects, and hence to sacrifice overall health. However, there was considerable heterogeneity between individuals in the importance attached to reducing a given health inequality, and in all questions the responses ranged from no targeting at all to targeting that results in less overall benefits for both groups. The nature and strength of an individual's preferences are often sensitive to what inequalities exist and where they exist. Within the questions asked, there were stronger preferences for reducing life expectancy inequalities than long-term illness inequalities. It also seems that people are much keener to reduce inequalities defined by social class than they are to reduce identical inequalities defined by sex or smoking status. The median respondent was indifferent about people in the lowest and highest social classes living on average to be 75 and 80 respectively, or living to be 75.5 and 78 respectively. If this information were fed into the SWF to determine the level of inequality aversion, the implied equity weight at the margin for those in social class 5 relative to those in social class 1 would be 6.6. But when the groups are defined in terms of sex, the median preference is to favour no targeting of men at all, so that the equity weight for men relative to women is 1.0.

Responses to the fourth interview question can be used to determine whether one group is seen to be more deserving than another. The results suggest that the weight given to a marginal health improvement for someone who has not cared for their health is about half (0.45) as much as that for someone who has cared for their health. These weights can then be applied to the responses to the question where an inequality in health exists between smokers and non-smokers, and which the smokers are to some extent responsible for. From responses to this study, the relative weight given to a marginal health improvement to a smoker in poorer health relative to a non-smoker in better health could be as low as 0.43 (on the assumption that the poorer health of smokers is entirely their responsibility).

The results from the postal survey are broadly in line with those from the interviews – people are concerned about inequalities in health, the perceived level of responsibility is seen as relevant, how health is defined matters, and the groups across which the inequalities exist also matter. But there were also some differences between the modes of administration. In particular, respondents to the postal questionnaire were, on average, less concerned than interviewees about health inequalities.

We examined inequalities between the sexes using a small focus group study of a stratified sample of the general public, in which two groups of about six men and two groups of about six women were given some basic facts about health inequalities between men and women and asked to comment on their possible causes and how important they thought it was to remedy them (Milborrow *et al.* 2003). The central piece of information given to the groups was that on average women live five years longer than men. In general, among the York citizens who participated in the study, women were willing to sacrifice life expectancy for their own sex in order to achieve gains for men, whereas men appeared to accept the inequality. Analysis of the qualitative data indicates that the reasons for these findings are complex. There is some suggestion that women are motivated by altruism, and are acting against their own self-interest. This is consistent with the view that women and men have different moral orientations, and that women display greater empathy with the situation of others than men do (see Gilligan 1993). However, some of the respondents (both male and female) articulated a more self-interested motivation, namely a desire to prolong the length of time that partners would have together, an objective that would be served by reducing inequalities in health between the sexes. Our sample was small and not representative of the population as a whole, so these observations should be seen as no more than tentative.

WHAT OTHER PEOPLE THINK

One of the authors (AW) has subsequently collected data from convenience samples (mostly health professionals) using three related questionnaires derived from all of this development work. One of these is shown in the appendix (see p. 81). The data are presented in the following tables, the first of which reports the data derived from the questionnaire in the appendix.

The responses in Table 3.1 can be interpreted as follows. Those choosing option A but then the programme offering three extra years to the better off and one extra year to the worse off are in favour of making the inequality greater. Those who choose policy A throughout are content to leave the existing inequality in lifetime health as it is, and/or are more concerned to equalize *gains*. Then we come to a group of responses which manifest some aversion to inequality, but only when the better off get some gains too. In the first case (A + 1&3) the total gain of four years is divided one to the better off and three to the worse off, and is preferred to two each. The other three responses in this group manifest a stronger aversion to inequality in outcomes, since the total amount of gain is diminishing, and the last response in this group (A + 1&1.5) indicates that some people would be willing to sacrifice one for the better off even if the gain to the worse off were lower (at 1.5) than it would have been if the 2&2 option had been chosen. The final group of responses includes those who initially chose B, and who subsequently indicated how much of a sacrifice in total gain they would be willing to accept in the pursuit of greater equality in the final distribution of life years. At the top are those who would give all four extra years to the worse off, but would abandon this targeting if any sacrifice in total health were involved. The subsequent rows show those who would make such a sacrifice, with the extreme case (B + 0&1.5) being those who would still give everything to the worse off even though both they and the better off would be worse off than under option A (that is, 2&2). For these respondents the pursuit of greater inequality is worth a big sacrifice.

Table 3.1 Inequalities in life expectancy between the social classes: results from various convenience samples

Would favour social class 1	
A + 3&1	16
NEUTRAL	
A + A	72
Would favour social class 5 but class 1 should benefit too	
A + 1&3	27
A + 1&2.5	6
A + 1&2	6
A + 1&1.5	17
Would favour social class 5 even if class 1 get nothing	
B + A	22
B + 0&3.5	24
B + 0&3	105
B + 0&2.5	76
B + 0&2	13
B + 0&1.5	32
TOTAL	**416**

Median respondent is in the shaded cell, and is willing to sacrifice two extra years for SC1 to get one extra year for SC5

Respondents

Birmingham public health	73
Italian health economists	51
Spanish health care personnel	48
Dutch/Flemish health economists	47
Australian public health	39
Dutch MDM forum	36
NZ Public health trainees	27
York health economics students	25
European philosophers forum	22
Dutch HTA	21
ISPOR workshop	14
York economics department	13

Concentrating now on the substance of Table 3.1, it transpires that the median respondent[2] prefers a programme that offers three extra years to social class 5 (and nothing to social class 1) over a programme which offers them two extra years each. Based on this, the equity weight at the initial point for a social class 5 person relative to a social class 1 person is 2.8 (much lower than the 6.6 derived from the general population). Exploring possible reasons for such differences is an important future research task.

Table 3.2 presents results for the same sized inequality in life expectancy, but now between smokers and non-smokers. It will be observed that the pattern of responses is entirely different. Roughly half of the respondents would do nothing to reduce this inequality, with the rest split equally between those who would favour the smokers and those who would favour the non-smokers. Incidentally, where it has been possible to separate the responses of current smokers, ex-smokers and never smokers, the median opinion in each subgroup is the same as for the group as a whole.

Finally, we come to the data on attitudes towards inequalities in life expectancy between the sexes. The data in Table 3.3 show a rather strange phenomenon. There is the same bimodal distribution of responses for respondents of each sex, so that the median (which is the same for each sex) falls in a relatively underpopulated part of the distribution. But although the largest single response is the 'neutral' one, two thirds of respondents would favour males to some extent, so the rather cautious views of the median respondent may well be the best basis for public policy.

Two messages stand out from these data. The first is that inequalities of the same magnitude were regarded in very different ways depending on their nature. Not all inequalities are equally inequitable (and perhaps some are not inequitable at all!). The second is that we need to know whether the views of the health professionals who form these convenience samples conform to the views of the general public.

WHERE DO WE GO FROM HERE?

From what has already been said it will be obvious that we see an important role for empirical research in helping bodies such as NICE formulate their position on matters of equity. NICE has to weigh the quantitative importance of the different objectives as they bear on the actual situation with their particular contexts. This means that it needs to have some idea of the trade-offs that would be acceptable to

Table 3.2 Inequalities in life expectancy between smokers and non-smokers: results from various convenience samples

Would favour non-smokers	
A + 3&1	59

NEUTRAL	
A + A	97

Would favour smokers but non-smokers should benefit too	
A + 1&3	5
A + 1&2.5	3
A + 1&2	0
A + 1&1.5	0

Would favour smokers even if non-smokers get nothing	
B + A	5
B + 0&3.5	8
B + 0&3	18
B + 0&2.5	14
B + 0&2	0
B + 0&1.5	0
TOTAL	**214**

Median respondent is in the shaded cell, and would not do anything to reduce this inequality

Respondents
Birmingham public health	74
Spanish health care personnel	49
Australian public health	39
Dutch MDM forum	38
York economics department	14

the general public, and apply these in a consistent manner from case to case.

The use of the SWF highlights the key parameters that need to be estimated, allowing systematic surveys of the general population.

Table 3.3 Inequalities in life expectancy between the sexes – by the sex of the respondents: results from various convenience samples

Respondent	Male	Female
Would favour females		
A + 3&1	1	7
NEUTRAL		
A + A	**45**	**47**
Would favour males but females should benefit too		
A + 1&3	13	11
A + 1&2.5	6	1
A + 1&2	0	1
A + 1&1.5	1	5
Would favour males even if females get nothing		
B + A	12	5
B + 0&3.5	8	4
B + 0&3	**17**	**28**
B + 0&2.5	12	17
B + 0&2	4	2
B + 0&1.5	8	4
TOTAL	**127**	**132**

Median respondent is in the shaded cell, but the median falls between two modes each in bold type in a bimodal distribution for both sexes!

Respondents

Birmingham public health	72 (M 28 : F 44)
Spanish health care personnel	48 (M 29 : F 19)
Australian public health	39 (M 15 : F 24)
Dutch MDM forum	38 (M 15 : F 23)
ISPOR workshop	31 (M 20 : F 11)
International course 2003	18 (M 11 : F 7)
York economics department	13 (M 9 : F 4)

But there are many complexities here which have so far only been partially explored. One such complexity is the very nature and stability of people's preferences. It is now widely recognized that preferences of the kind referred to here can be highly sensitive to such factors as the wording of the question and the mode of administration. In the ESRC study referred to above, we have evidence that the presence of an interviewer may affect a respondent's answers so that they appear more concerned about inequalities in health than is the case when the questionnaire is completed in private. This is not to say that postal surveys are to be preferred. In fact, we would argue precisely the opposite since a postal survey provides no opportunity to understand anything about the reasoning behind people's preferences – and this is something that is vital if we are to use stated preferences to inform policy. So, we need to develop methods that allow us to understand more about preferences, while at the same time influencing them less.

Because it is easier for people to understand, the elicitation of aversion to inequality has hitherto focused on life expectancy as the relevant statistic. But we think that it should really be focused on *quality-adjusted* life expectancy, even though this is likely to make things a lot more complicated. There is some evidence that people view the two differently, and may even have views that are sensitive to the particular element in health-related quality of life (HRQL) that is generating the greatest differences between groups (for instance, whether it is differences in pain or differences in mobility).

It is already clear that people have different views on inequalities depending on their cause and the subgroups that are being compared. It is to be expected that people would be more averse to large inequalities than to small ones, and there may be a threshold effect below which people would not bother to do anything at all about them.

Where more than one equity principle is in play simultaneously, we shall have to contend with equity-equity trade-offs as well as equity-efficiency trade-offs. Thus the problem of deriving equity weights will become even more complex, especially if there is interaction between them.

This multiplicity of considerations raises another important issue. In the research reported above we have been concerned with population subgroups, which are defined in terms of one attribute at a time (e.g. social class, or smoking status). Can we infer from this what the relative weight should be between a smoker from social class 1 vs. a non-smoker from social class 5? It may be possible to find some functional relationship between the single attribute weights to derive the multi-attribute weights, making them more policy relevant. But this is unlikely to be straightforward, and will doubtless require further empirical work to directly elicit public opinions on these more complex cases.

Finally, when people assess inequalities in *health*, they may also be taking into account other inequalities, such as those in socio-economic opportunities, which they may regard either as moderating the importance of health inequalities or exacerbating them. This opens up a further area of research regarding the applicability of the FIA to overall well-being, where health will be but one of the elements to be weighed in the assessment of social welfare.

CONCLUSIONS

In our analysis we have focused on the generation of equity weights by eliciting people's subjective trade-offs between different objectives. Giving a central role to the efficiency costs of various equity positions is an important feature, since it directs attention to the fact that, once you adopt objectives other than that of maximizing the health of the whole community, you are bound to find yourself making decisions in which the average health of the population is lower than it could have been. This may well be justifiable, but the reasoning needs to be explicit and deliberate, not implicit and inadvertent.

As was stated at the outset, NICE does not formulate the problem in terms of equity weights, but in terms of cost per QALY thresholds, above which they will not recommend the adoption of a technology. This is not a serious conceptual problem, since we have shown that equity weights can be mapped onto such thresholds quite directly. To say that a health gain to A is twice as valuable (in terms of social welfare) as the same health gain to B is tantamount to saying that it would be worth spending twice as much to provide that health gain for A as it would be worth spending for the same health gain for B. Thus the obvious way for NICE to incorporate equity considerations into its decisions is to establish an explicit 'tariff' of threshold adjustments according to the weight that it attaches to each specific equity consideration. In this manner it can be both transparent and consistent.

The argument of this chapter is that if bodies such as NICE are to reflect the values of the people they serve, they need to find out what those values are in this rather difficult territory. Equity arguments are not normally conducted in quantitative terms, and it is going to take some careful exploratory research to find reliable ways of doing this and generating data that can be used with confidence in public decision-making. However, although this is likely to be a difficult enterprise, we have sought to show here that we are not starting from scratch.

APPENDIX: TRADE-OFF QUESTIONNAIRE CONCERNING SOCIAL CLASS INEQUALITIES

AVERAGE LIFE EXPECTANCY

As you might know, average life expectancy differs by social class. There are differences between people in social class 1 (for example, doctors and lawyers) and people in social class 5 (for example, road-sweepers and cleaners). These two groups are more or less equal in size (they each make up about 7% of the population).

Whilst actual life expectancy varies between individuals, on average people in social class 1 live to be **75** and in social class 5 they live to be **70**.

Imagine that you are asked to choose between two programmes which will increase average life expectancy. Both programmes cost the same.

In the two graphs below the light coloured part shows average life expectancy, and the dark coloured part shows the increase in life expectancy. There is a separate graph for each of the programmes.

As you can see, Programme A is aimed at both social classes and Programme B is aimed only at social class 5.

Please indicate whether you would choose A or B by ticking one box.

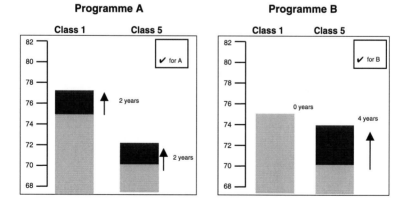

If you chose A, please go to 'Follow-up Sheet A'.

If you chose B, please go to 'Follow-up Sheet B'.

FOLLOW-UP SHEET A

For each of the five choices below, please tick one box to indicate whether you would still choose Programme A, or whether you would now choose Programme B.

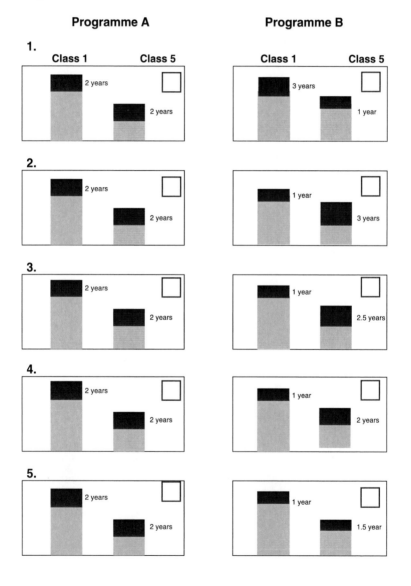

FOLLOW-UP SHEET B

What would your view be if it turned out that Programme B is less effective than we had first thought, and the increase in life expectancy for social class 5 is as shown below. For each of the five choices, please tick one box to indicate whether you would still choose B, or whether you would now choose A.

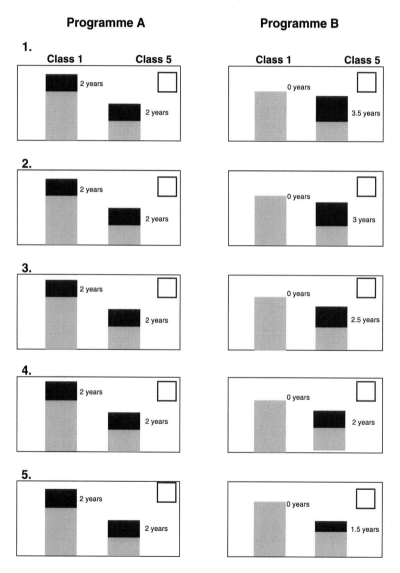

DISCUSSION
John Hutton

The aim of the chapter is to explore the ways in which equity considerations might be explicitly and quantitatively incorporated into the decision-making processes of priority-setting bodies such as NICE. The authors identify two major concepts within the discussion of distributive justice – egalitarianism and desert – both of which could lead to individuals with equal capacity to benefit from a health intervention being treated differently. They favour a version of the FIA to reducing inequalities in quality-adjusted lifetime health experience, which they think will fit well with NICE's preferred approach to measurement of overall health gain. They are less enamoured of the 'rule of rescue' approach, which they feel is inappropriate for a body making evidence-based judgments on behalf of society. Both these approaches lead to a reduction in overall health gain in order to reduce inequality. The rule of rescue is felt to involve too great a sacrifice in health benefits to others, given the small impact on the target group.

Empirical work with the general public has shown support for the 'rule of rescue', equalization of lifetime health, and health maximization. There is a general willingness to sacrifice total health gain in order to reduce inequality, but there are heterogeneous views on the 'desert' of different groups. There was more support for reducing inequalities attributed to social class differences than to those to which the behaviour of the individual might have contributed (e.g. smokers). The median response was that the reduction of health inequalities between the sexes should not be given priority, but views on this were varied between groups of respondents.

From the exploratory research, the authors identify the complexities of deriving a community-based set of equity weights, as they must simultaneously incorporate views on willingness to sacrifice health gain for reduced inequality, the deservedness of different groups, and the types of inequality to be addressed. Although unwilling to draw firm policy guidelines from the exploratory research, they feel that enough has been learnt from this to embark on a more comprehensive national research agenda, perhaps along the lines of the MVH study on social valuation of health states.

The characterization of the issues and the analytical approach of the chapter are very sound, and, apart from concerns about the

use of stated preference methods, which the authors acknowledge, what they propose will certainly lead to clarification of
thinking and increased knowledge of what people really think.
There are concerns about the practicality of using such an
approach in decision-making, both in terms of collecting the
information on the beneficiaries of treatment and in allocating
resources to the prioritized groups.

So far as NICE is concerned, it currently considers equity issues
in the context of a policy framework laid down by the health min-
istry. NICE has a set of criteria that influences the topics it
addresses, one of which is the contribution to specific government
initiatives, such as tackling inequalities. It has, furthermore, established a Citizens' Council that seeks to take direct account of the
views of the general public. However, it is a big step to go from this
position to advocating the use of equity-weighted QALYs to
decide which treatments are offered and to whom.

Experience indicates that there are few diseases in which the
sufferers are homogeneous in their social characteristics. Some
can be described as diseases of old age, perhaps, and some are
gender-specific. Few diseases are caused solely by the behaviour of
those suffering from them. Currently NICE considers health technologies individually, and tries to identify the subgroup of patients
most likely to receive sufficient benefit to justify the use of the
resources. The identification is by capacity to benefit in line with
the health maximization approach, but is tempered by ad hoc
introduction of other considerations in some cases. Clarification
and quantification might be helpful in improving the consistency
of the application of non-efficiency factors, but it would be difficult to label *technologies* as egalitarian or otherwise. If desert is
judged at the individual level, the person who decides whether to
offer treatment will be faced with an even more difficult task than
at present. Systematic lengthening of waiting times for treatment
for those in higher income groups, for example, would raise a set
of additional equity issues involving use of private medicine.

Partly for these reasons, previous policy initiatives to reduce
health inequalities have targeted resources at geographical areas
thought to contain a preponderance of disadvantaged people (see
Chapter 8). The intention is to make available greater quantities of
potentially beneficial treatments to those with the poorest health,
but the targeting is not perfect. Perhaps the main benefit of the
quantification of the public's views on the equity-efficiency trade-
off would be to test the validity of the professionally and politically

driven initiatives currently in operation. This implies that the range of health technologies which NICE is asked to appraise should include organizational issues as well as those directly concerned with treatment. Such appraisals would place equity issues to the fore, as the intended output measure is reduction in inequality. The current importance of NICE may be a useful focus for generating support for further empirical work. The feasibility and desirability of micro-weighting for equity in appraisals of treatments remains to be established.

NOTES

1   As will be evident from the text, this work would not have been possible without the contributions of Richard Cookson, Wendy Milberrow and Rebecca Shaw, not to mention all the people who provided raw material in our interviews and surveys. We hope that what we have made of all this meets with their approval.
2   The location of the median in these tables is a bit complicated, because the manifested degree of inequality aversion is not monotonically increasing by row from top to bottom. In fact, the monotonically increasing order by row number is: 1, 2, 7, 3, 8, 9, 4, 10, 5, (6 or 11), 12. The reason why rows 6 and 11 are bracketed together is that it is not clear whether a preference for 1&1.5 over 2&2 is more or less inequality averse than a preference for 0&3 over 2&2. Fortunately, in the data collected so far, these responses have been a long way from the median position.

REFERENCES

Cookson, R. and Dolan, P. (1999) Public views on health care rationing: a group discussion study, *Health Policy*, 49: 63–74.
Cookson, R. and Dolan, P. (2000) Rationing health care: what philosophers and the public think, *Journal of Medical Ethics*, 26: 323–9.
DHSS (Department of Health and Social Security) (1980) *Inequalities in Health: Report of a Working Group*. London: HMSO.
Dolan, P. and Tsuchiya, A. (2003) The social welfare function and individual responsibility: some theoretical issues and empirical evidence from health. Discussion paper, Sheffield Health Economics Group.
Dolan, P., Cookson, R. and Ferguson, B. (1999) The effect of group discussions on the public's view regarding priorities in health care, *British Medical Journal*, 318: 916–19.
Dolan, P., Tsuchiya, A., Smith, P., Shaw, R. and Williams, A. (2002) Determining the parameters in a social welfare function using stated preference data: an application to health. Discussion Paper, Sheffield Health Economics Group.

Dolan, P., Shaw, R., Tsuchiya, A. and Williams, A. (2004) QALY maximisation and people's preferences: a systematic review of the literature, *Health Economics*, forthcoming.

Gilligan, C. (1993). *In a Different Voice*. London: Harvard University Press.

Glover, J. (1977) *Causing Death and Saving Lives*. Harmondsworth: Penguin.

Harris, J. (1985) *The Value of Life*. London: Routledge.

Independent Inquiry into Inequalities in Health (1998) *Independent Inquiry into Inequalities in Health*. London: The Stationery Office.

McKie, J. and Richardson, J. (2003) The rule of rescue, *Social Science and Medicine*, 56: 2407–19.

Milborrow, W., Tsuchiya, A. and Williams, A. (2003) A fair innings between the sexes: what men say and what women say. Paper presented at the Health Economists' Study Group, Canterbury.

NICE (2002) *Report of the First Meeting of the NICE Citizens Council: Determining Clinical Need*, http://www.nice.org.uk/pdf/ FINALNICEFirstMeeting_FINALReport.pdf.

NICE (2003) *Guide to the Methods of Technology Appraisal: Draft for Consultation*. http://www.nice.org.uk/pdf/methodologyconsultationdraftfinal. pdf.

Shaw, R., Dolan, P., Tsuchiya, A., Williams, A., Smith, P. and Burrows, R. (2001) *Development of a Questionnaire to Elicit People's Preferences Regarding Health Inequalities*, occasional paper. University of York: Centre for Health Economics.

Tsuchiya, A. (2000) QALYs and ageism: philosophical theories and age weighting, *Health Economics*, 9(1): 57–68.

Tsuchiya, A. and Williams, A. (2004) A 'fair innings' between the sexes: are men being treated inequitably? *Social Science and Medicine*, forthcoming.

Williams, A. (1997) Intergenerational equity: an exploration of the 'fair innings' argument, *Health Economics*, 6: 117–32.

4

USING LONGITUDINAL DATA TO INVESTIGATE SOCIOECONOMIC INEQUALITY IN HEALTH

Andrew Jones and Nigel Rice

INTRODUCTION

Inequalities in health are a fundamental policy concern in most countries. Yet, in spite of numerous initiatives designed to address the issue, health inequalities remain a remarkably persistent and indeed growing policy problem. A fundamental requirement for developing policy in this domain is a sound understanding of the processes that contribute to the creation of health inequalities. A great deal of academic research effort has therefore focused on measuring and identifying the nature of inequalities in health and has speculated on the form policy initiatives may take to help reduce such inequalities. The disciplines of public health and epidemiology have contributed greatly to this end.

Health economics has also been at the forefront of developing analytic tools for the measurement and explanation of socioeconomic inequalities in health. The aim of this chapter is to highlight the distinct contributions made by economists to the measurement and explanation of socioeconomic inequalities in health, and to point towards areas of potential future research that will help to illuminate the nature and composition of health inequalities. We will concentrate on the central role that income plays, both as an instrument in the measurement of health inequalities, and as a determinant of health and inequality in health.

To date, analytic efforts have usually been constrained by the limited availability of data. Typically these are available only in the form of one-off cross-sectional surveys. While offering some valuable insights, such surveys cannot address a fundamental characteristic of health inequalities: that they appear to persist over time, in spite of policies aimed at promoting equal access and combating social exclusion. It is therefore clear that attention must be paid to the dynamics of health and their relation to socioeconomic characteristics. Increasingly, countries are implementing longitudinal surveys of individuals and households that offer the prospect of new insights into the dynamics of inequalities. Such analysis is far from straightforward, and often requires the careful deployment of advanced econometric techniques. This chapter therefore provides an overview of econometric methods for the analysis of health inequalities and health mobility when such longitudinal data are available.

In particular, we concentrate on the long-running *ECuity Project*, which has pioneered the use of economic tools to measure inequality and inequity in the financing and delivery of health care and in the distribution of health within the population. The ECuity Project has recently entered a new phase, 'ECuity III'. The methodology of the ECuity III Project will be built around the analysis of longitudinal data: both the European Community Household Panel (ECHP) and other national datasets such as the British Household Panel Survey (BHPS). This will entail panel data econometric analysis of the impact of income on health, the dynamics of health, the impact of health on earnings and labour market outcomes such as early retirement, and on the utilization of health care. Results from these econometric analyses will form the basis for the measurement and explanation of socioeconomic inequalities. The chapter highlights recent innovations in these methods.

Although the methods are relevant to analysis of longitudinal survey data in any setting, we focus on the UK experience, where health inequalities have assumed an especially high policy priority. In spite of the nation's increased prosperity, there remain striking inequalities in health across geographical areas and between socioeconomic groups within society, and evidence suggests that such inequalities are widening. Concern over the level of health inequalities prompted the commission of Sir Donald Acheson's *Independent Inquiry into Inequalities in Health* (Acheson 1998). This summarized evidence about the scale and nature of health inequalities and formed the foundation of subsequent policy initiatives aimed at their amelioration. Targeting groups most at risk in an attempt to tackle such inequalities has been stated as a top priority of the government (Department of Health 2002).

The NHS Plan (Department of Health 2000) has emphasized the commitment to reduce inequalities in health by providing extra funding for the National Health Service (NHS). Additional resources are being directed to areas of greatest need through improved resource allocation mechanisms and monies ring-fenced specifically for the reduction of health inequalities. Linked to these are national targets for 2010 to reduce the gap in infant mortality across social class groups and to raise life expectancy in the most disadvantaged areas faster than elsewhere. Moreover, *Tackling Health Inequalities: A Programme for Action* (Department of Health 2003) states the need to improve the health of the poorest 30–40 per cent of the population if significant reductions in health inequalities are to be achieved. Further efforts to tackle inequalities in health have been taken, in part, through policy initiatives such as increasing the minimum wage, welfare and benefit reforms, transport and housing improvements, Sure Start and Neighbourhood Renewal Schemes. These policies indicate a commitment on behalf of the government to a cross-departmental perspective to reducing health inequalities. Indeed, the recent review *Tackling Health Inequalities* (Department of Health 2002) seeks to place health inequalities at the heart of every key public service and recognizes the need for concerted action across government and with other sectors.

Further concerns over the level of inequalities in health have been expressed in the '*Wanless Report*', *Securing Our Future Health: Taking a Long-Term View* (Wanless 2002). In his review of future health care resource requirements, Wanless calls for a better understanding of the role of income and other socioeconomic inequalities in explaining observed differences in health outcomes and the subsequent use of health care. It is noted that health inequalities affect resource requirements for health and social care, but knowledge of how socioeconomic need and health need are related is incomplete.

The organization of the chapter is as follows. The next section introduces concepts of measurement appropriate for income-related health inequalities. Some of the econometric methods used to analyse longitudinal data are then outlined, and some illustrative results presented. We conclude with some brief comments on future prospects in this domain.

MEASUREMENT OF INCOME-RELATED INEQUALITY

Concentration and Gini indices

In order to measure socioeconomic or income-related inequality in health, economists have borrowed tools from the income inequality literature. Foremost among these is the health concentration index, which provides a measure of relative income-related health inequality (Wagstaff *et al.* 1989).

The health concentration index is derived from the health concentration curve, which is illustrated in Figure 4.1. The sample of interest is ranked by socioeconomic status, so if income is used as the relevant ranking variable, the horizontal axis begins with the poorest individual in society and progresses through the income distribution up to the very richest individual in society. This relative income rank is then plotted against the cumulative proportion of health on the vertical axis. This assumes that a cardinal measure of health is available, and can be compared and aggregated across individuals. The 45° line shows the line of perfect equality, in which case shares of population health are proportional to income, such that the poorest 20 per cent of individuals receive 20 per cent of the available health in the population and so on. In reality there is likely to be pro-rich inequality in the distribution of health, and this is illustrated by the convex curve on the figure – the concentration curve. In the example shown, the poorest 20 per cent of income earners receive less than 20 per cent of the health available. So the fact that the concentration curve lies below the line of perfect equality indicates that there is pro-rich inequality in health. The size of this inequality can be

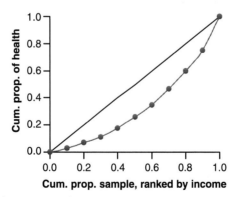

Figure 4.1   The concentration curve

summarized by the health concentration index (C), which is given by twice the lens-shaped area between the concentration curve and the 45° line.

There are various ways of expressing the concentration index (C) algebraically. The one that is most convenient for our purposes is

$$C = \frac{2}{\mu} \sum_{i=1}^{N} (y_i - \mu)(R_i - \frac{1}{2}) = \frac{2}{\mu} \, \text{cov}(y_i, R_i)$$

This shows that the value of the concentration index is equal to the covariance between individual health (y) and the individual's relative rank (R), scaled by the mean of health in the population (μ). Then the whole expression is multiplied by 2, to ensure the concentration index lies between −1 and +1. Writing the concentration index in this way emphasizes that it is an indicator of the degree of association between an individual's level of health and their relative position in the income distribution. Concentration indices are sometimes criticized for being hard to interpret: what does a value of, say, 0.04 mean? A recent contribution by Koolman and van Doorslaer (2004) helps to clarify the situation. They show that, if the concentration index is interpreted in terms of a hypothetical linear redistribution from rich to poor, it can be given a Robin Hood-type interpretation. This interpretation implies that 75 times the concentration index is the percentage of total y that would have to be redistributed from individuals in the richest half to individuals in the poorest half of the population to achieve an equal distribution

Recent work by Bommier and Stechklov (2002) argues that concentration curves, and by implication the concentration index, are a more appropriate way to measure socioeconomic inequality in health than inequality indices derived from social welfare functions that have health and income as arguments. This is the case if equity is defined according to a social justice approach that defines 'the health distribution in the ideal equitable society as one where access to health has not been determined by socioeconomic status or income' (Bommier and Stechklov 2002: 502).

Socioeconomic inequality in health is cited widely as a concern for health policymakers. However, it may not be the whole story. Recent work at the World Health Organization (WHO) through their Evidence for Health Policy programme has argued that policymakers should also be concerned about other sources of inequality, and that measurement should focus on total health inequality (Gakidou *et al.* 2000). This can be analysed using health Lorenz curves and inequality can be measured using the Gini coefficient of health inequality (Le Grand 1989; Wagstaff *et al.* 1991). The attraction of this approach is that there is a direct relationship between the concentration index and the Gini coefficient for health: the concentration index is proportional to the Gini coefficient, where the factor of proportionality is given by the ratio between the correlation coefficient for health and income rank and the correlation coefficient between health and health rank (Kakwani 1980; van Doorslaer and Jones 2003). This means that it is easy to move between these measures of socioeconomic and pure health inequality.

The inequality literature makes a distinction between partial orderings, based on Lorenz or concentration curves, and complete orderings, based on index numbers such as the Gini and concentration indices. A partial ordering means that some, but not all, combinations of distributions can be ranked unambiguously. The ambiguity arises if the Lorenz or concentration curves for two distributions cross each other. In order to obtain a complete ordering of distributions, Gini coefficients and concentration indices embed particular normative judgements about the weight given to individuals at different points in the income distribution and, hence, they embody a particular degree of inequality aversion. Sensitivity of the results to inequality aversion can be assessed by using extended Gini or concentration indices (Yitzhaki 1983; Lerman and Yitzhaki 1984; Wagstaff 2002). These add an extra parameter that can range from inequality neutrality (no concern for inequality) to extreme inequality aversion (Rawlsian lexi-min).

Gini and concentration indices are measures of relative inequality and do not address the equity-efficiency trade-off. This trade-off can be captured by generalized Lorenz or concentration curves. These multiply the Lorenz or concentration curve by the absolute level of health. A classic result from the income equality literature – the Kakwani-Kolm-Shorrocks theorem – shows that generalized Lorenz dominance is equivalent to a distribution having a greater level of social welfare for any welfare function that is increasing and concave in income. The generalized concentration index, $\mu(1 - C)$, gives a single index that captures the trade-off between the mean of the distribution (μ) and the level of inequality. This can be combined with different degrees of inequality aversion, through the extended concentration index, to give what Wagstaff (2002) calls an index of health achievement. This index summarizes the equity-efficiency trade-off for different degrees of inequality aversion.

The following analysis assumes that a cardinal measure of health is available. This is relatively straightforward for indicators of illness, such as the presence of chronic conditions, as the concentration index or Gini coefficient can be based on the headcount of the number of individuals experiencing the illness. It is more difficult when health is measured using self-reported subjective scales. Self-assessed health (SAH) is widely available in many general population surveys and has been used extensively in the ECuity Project. The problem with this measure is that respondents are asked to describe their health in ordered categories and the variable is inherently ordinal rather than cardinal. In the past, researchers have dealt with ordinal measures of health either by dichotomizing the variable so that individuals are described as either healthy or non-healthy, or by imposing some sort of scaling assumption. The problem with the former is that information is lost and not all of the health variation contained in the original SAH variable is used. Evidence shows that comparisons of inequality over time or across populations may be sensitive because the results differ depending on the choice of the cut-point between healthy and non-healthy. A variety of methods have been used to re-scale the ordinal measure of health into a cardinal measure.

Early work in the ECuity Project imposed a lognormal distribution on self-assessed health (SAH). More recently, external information (such as the average level of health utility within categories of self-assessed health (SAH)) has been used in the re-scaling. A third approach is to adopt an appropriate econometric specification, such as the ordered probit model, and use the predictions from this model as a scaled measure of individual health.

Van Doorslaer and Jones (2003) suggest an approach that combines the use of external information with the ordered probit model. This relies on having a dataset that includes both self-assessed health (SAH) and a cardinal index of health: in their case the Canadian National Population Health Survey (NPHS), which includes SAH and the McMaster health utility index (HUI). This is used to construct a mapping from HUI to SAH. On the assumption that there is a systematic relationship between the two measures of health – such that those at the bottom of the distribution of SAH will also be those at the bottom of the distribution of health utility – it is possible to scale the cut-points for categories of SAH using health utility values. These cut-points can then be incorporated into the ordered probit model and self-assessed health (SAH) can be estimated as an interval regression, where the values of the cut-points are treated as known. The attraction of this approach is that predictions from the interval regression model are on the same scale as health utility.

Figure 4.2, taken from van Doorslaer and Koolman (2002), illustrates an international comparison of concentration indices for socioeconomic inequality in health based on the Europanel (ECHP) data. These are calculated using the interval regression method of scaling self-assessed health (SAH). The horizontal axis shows the level of income inequality measured by the Gini coefficient for log income, while the vertical axis shows health inequality measured by the concentration index. The Netherlands (NL) and Germany (DE) have the lowest levels of socioeconomic inequality in health, while Portugal (PT) stands out as having both the highest levels of

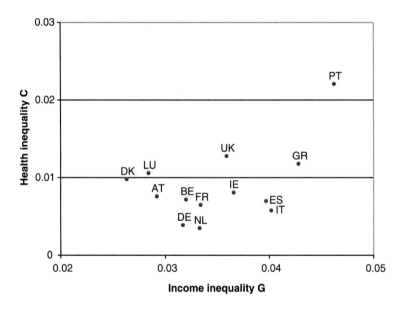

Figure 4.2   Income and health inequality in Europe
Source: van Doorslaer and Koolman (2002)

Key

AT: AUSTRIA	IE: IRELAND
BE: BELGIUM	IT: ITALY
DE: GERMANY	LU: LUXEMBOURG
DK: DENMARK	NL: THE NETHERLANDS
ES: SPAIN	PT: PORTUGAL
FR: FRANCE	UK: UNITED KINGDOM
GR: GREECE	

income inequality and of socioeconomic inequality in health. These numbers summarize international differences in the overall level of socioeconomic inequality in health as measured by the association between health and income rank. The story can be taken further by decomposing the concentration index into its component parts.

Decomposing inequality indices

Like the Gini coefficient of income inequality, the concentration index has the attraction, that it can be decomposed by factors (Rao 1969; Kakwani 1980). For example, this property has been used in the past to decompose the concentration index for health care financing into different sources of health care payments such as taxation, social insurance contributions, user charges etc. A recent paper by Wagstaff *et al.* (2003) exploits the result that if a reduced form of demand for health equation is additively separable,

$$y_i = a + \sum_k \beta_k x_{ki} + \varepsilon_i,$$

then, because the concentration index is additively decomposable – which stems from the fact that the covariance of a linear combination is equal to the linear combination of covariances – the overall concentration index for health can be written as follows:

$$C = \sum_k (\beta_k \bar{x}_k / \mu) C_k + GC_\varepsilon / \mu = C_{\hat{y}} + GC_\varepsilon / \mu$$

This has the convenient form that C can be split into two parts. The first term can be thought of as the explained component ($C_{\hat{y}}$) and the second term as the unexplained component. Within the explained component there is a contribution for each of the regressors (X) and this is made up of the product of two terms. The first term is the elasticity of health with respect to that variable (e.g. the income elasticity of health), and the second term is the concentration index of that variable (e.g. in the case of income this would be the Gini coefficient).

Figure 4.3 shows the decomposition of concentration indices based on the 1996 ECHP, and is taken from van Doorslaer and Koolman (2002). The length of the horizontal bars indicates the overall size of the concentration index for each country, and the

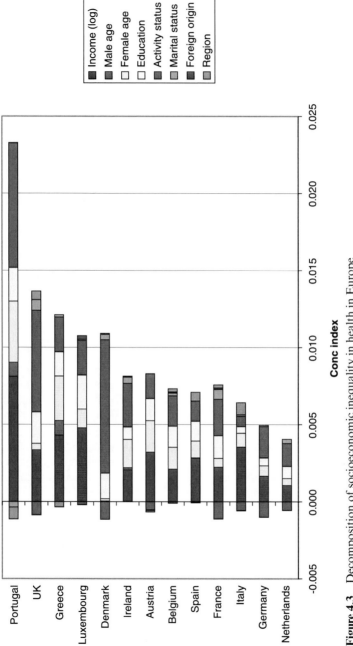

Figure 4.3 Decomposition of socioeconomic inequality in health in Europe
Source: van Doorslaer and Koolman (2002)

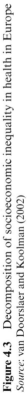

shaded blocks show the contribution of different groups of variables. One notable feature is that although income itself makes a sizeable contribution in most countries, it is only part of the story. Other sources of income-related inequality in health include variables such as activity status. In fact it is striking that, in Denmark, activity status explains the bulk of the association between health and income rank, with a negligible contribution from income itself.

Standardized concentration indices

The concentration index measures income-related inequality in health. This is not the same thing as inequity in health. For example, variations in health that are attributable to age and gender may be seen as unavoidable and hence legitimate sources of inequality. The same argument applies to measures of inequality in the use of health care (van Doorslaer *et al.* 2003). Usually, the horizontal version of the egalitarian principle is interpreted to require that people in equal need of care are treated equally, irrespective of characteristics such as income, place of residence, race etc. While the concentration index of medical care use (C_M) measures the degree of inequality in the use of medical care by income, it does not yet measure the degree of inequity. For any inequality to be interpretable as inequity, legitimate or need-determined inequality has to be taken into account.

There are two broad ways of standardizing distributions for differences in need: the direct and the indirect methods. The direct method proceeds by computing a concentration index for medical care use that would emerge if each individual had the same need characteristics as the population as a whole. Wagstaff *et al.* (1991) have used this procedure to compute what they call HI_{WVP} indices, which are essentially directly standardized concentration indices. More recently, Wagstaff and van Doorslaer (2000) have advocated the technique of indirect standardization for the measurement of so-called HI_{WV} indices on the grounds that it is computationally easier and does not rely on grouped data. A measure of the need for medical care is obtained for each individual as the predicted use from a regression on need indicators. This means that, in order to statistically equalize need for the groups or individuals to be compared, one is effectively using the average relationship between need and treatment for the sample as a whole as the vertical equity norm, and horizontal inequity is measured by systematic deviations from this norm by income level.

The issue of the role of explanatory models in the measurement of inequity deserves some further attention. Recently, some authors have drawn attention to the potential biases involved in these standardization procedures. First, the problem of determining which systematic variations in medical care use by income are 'needed' and therefore, in a sense, justifiable, and which are not, bears some resemblance to the problem of determining legitimate compensation in the risk adjustment literature. Schokkaert and van de Voorde (2000) have argued that while there is a difference between the positive exercise of *explaining* medical care expenditure (or use) and the normative issue of *justifying* medical expenditure (or use) differences, the results of the former exercise have relevance for the second. Drawing on the theory of fair compensation, they show that failure to include 'responsibility variables' (which *do not* need to be compensated for in the capitation formula) in the equation used for estimating the effect of 'compensation variables' (which *do* need to be compensated for) may give rise to omitted variable bias in the determination of the 'appropriate' capitations (or fair compensations). Their proposed remedy to this problem is to include the 'omitted variables' in the estimation equation but to 'neutralize' their impact by setting these variables equal to their means in the need-prediction equation. A similar argument to Schokkaert and van de Voorde was made and taken further by Gravelle (2003) in the context of the measurement of income-related inequality of health or health care. He uses an 'augmented partial concentration index' which is defined as the (directly) standardized concentration index, but controlling for income and other non-standardizing variables in the process. This can be obtained from the regression-based decomposition of the concentration index.

One important problem with measuring horizontal inequity and applying the decomposition analysis is that the dependent variable in health care demand models is typically specified as a non-linear function of the regressors: for example, in van Doorslaer *et al.* (2003) the empirical models of health care use are based on logistic, truncated and generalized negative binomial regression models, which are intrinsically non-linear. So long as the model is linear, then the Schokkaert and van de Voorde (2000) approach of estimating the linear regression and then neutralizing the non-need variables by setting them equal to their mean (or, in fact, any constant value) and the decomposition approach lead to the same measure of horizontal inequity (van Doorslaer *et al.*, 2003). This does not hold for a non-linear model, as the linear decomposition does not apply. However, it is possible to approximate the decomposition analysis. To do this, van Doorslaer *et al.* (2003) opted to use a linearized 'partial effects' representation for the decomposition. This has the advantage of being a linear additive model of actual utilization, but is only an approximation.

Measurement of inequality and mobility with panel data

Up to now we have focused on methods for the measurement and explanation of socioeconomic inequalities in health that have been designed for use with cross-sectional data. Jones and López Nicolás (2003) explore what more can be gained by using panel data. Again it is possible to borrow from the income inequality literature. Work on income mobility has focused on comparing the distribution of income using two perspectives: first of all a cross-sectional or short-run perspective and second a long-run perspective where income is aggregated over a series of periods. If an individual's income rank differs between the short run and the long run there is evidence of income mobility. One way of measuring this phenomenon is through the index of income mobility proposed by Shorrocks (1978).

The aim of the paper by Jones and López Nicolás (2003) is to apply the same principles to income-related health inequality. They show that the long-run concentration index can be written as the sum of a weighted average of short-run concentration indices plus a term that captures the covariance between levels of health and fluctuations in income rank over time. This differs from income inequality in that income-related health inequality can be either greater or smaller in the long run than the short run but, once again, these changes can be measured through an index of health-related income mobility which is based on the familiar tools of the concentration index. This mobility index can be decomposed using the contribution of different factors through a regression model for health and this is illustrated using the General Health Questionnaire (GHQ) measure of subjective well-being from the first nine waves of the BHPS. This shows that, after nine waves, the weighted average of short-run measures under-estimates the long-run measure by 15 per cent for men and 5 per cent for women.

The distinction between the short run and the long run will be of interest to policymakers whose ethical concern is with inequalities in long-run health. For example, the 'fair innings' perspective suggests that equity should be defined in terms of a person's lifetime experience of health (Williams and Cookson 2000: 1899). In practice, this lifetime experience could be measured using disability-adjusted life years (DALYs, Murray and Lopez 1996) or quality-adjusted life years (QALYs, Williams 1997).

PANEL DATA ECONOMETRIC ANALYSIS OF HEALTH

The previous section summarized recent innovations in the measurement and explanation of socioeconomic inequalities in health and concluded by showing the scope for using longitudinal data to learn more about the dynamics of health inequalities. This section turns to the estimation of regression models for health that also exploit the longitudinal dimension of panel data.

Empirical evidence on mobility in health

Empirical research into the extent and nature of inequalities in health has, to date, tended to rely on cross-sectional observations of the level of observed health within socioeconomic groups of interest. Cross-sectional information can, at best, provide a snapshot of the overall distribution of health at any particular point in time with respect to factors of interest such as income, employment status or social class. What it cannot provide is evidence on the intertemporal experience of health problems and how this may vary across different socioeconomic groups.

We have described methods to measure intertemporal mobility in income-related health inequalities based on the index of income mobility proposed by Shorrocks (1978). An empirical study aimed at incorporating a time dimension into the analysis of health inequalities is provided by Hauck and Rice (2003). The paper is concerned with the extent to which individuals move over time within the overall distribution of mental health. Mobility is then compared across socioeconomic groups. Interest focuses on both the level of observed mental illness and how mobile, over time, individuals are within their respective health distributions. Data from 11 waves of the BHPS are used.

As in Jones and López Nicolás (2003), the measure of mental health is based on the 12-item version of the GHQ. The GHQ is a self-administered screening test aimed at detecting psychiatric disorders that require clinical attention among respondents in community settings and non-psychiatric clinical settings. A Likert scale is used to form an overall score for each respondent based on summing

across the item-specific responses. This provides a variable ranging
from 0 (least problems) to 36 (most problems).

A simple description of mobility is presented for men and women
in Table 4.1. The correlations in GHQ scores across the 11 waves of
data show a clear pattern. As expected, waves closer together have, in
general, higher correlations than waves further apart. The highest
correlations occur in the cells adjacent to the lead diagonal. These
correlations then show a tendency to decrease as one moves further
away from the lead diagonal until a degree of levelling out occurs.

Table 4.1 Correlation matrices

Men

Wave	1	2	3	4	5	6	7	8	9	10	11
1	1.00										
2	.489	1.00									
3	.422	.531	1.00								
4	.388	.451	.524	1.00							
5	.383	.454	.484	.526	1.00						
6	.338	.393	.414	.471	.556	1.00					
7	.316	.348	.383	.455	.451	.532	1.00				
8	.328	.374	.385	.421	.436	.467	.525	1.00			
9	.315	.361	.373	.406	.392	.442	.465	.536	1.00		
10	.353	.359	.391	.404	.388	.409	.433	.455	.544	1.00	
11	.355	.351	.363	.401	.386	.392	.395	.441	.477	.538	1.00

Women

Wave	1	2	3	4	5	6	7	8	9	10	11
1	1.00										
2	.484	1.00									
3	.444	.506	1.00								
4	.395	.438	.516	1.00							
5	.363	.386	.408	.502	1.00						
6	.357	.370	.387	.435	.470	1.00					
7	.332	.311	.322	.368	.435	.456	1.00				
8	.322	.302	.348	.393	.402	.444	.525	1.00			
9	.327	.328	.352	.352	.391	.411	.448	.504	1.00		
10	.331	.309	.354	.331	.334	.370	.387	.463	.521	1.00	
11	.324	.325	.315	.323	.329	.347	.355	.422	.464	.518	1.00

Source: Hauck and Rice (2003)

The off-diagonal correlations vary between 0.315 and 0.556 for men and 0.302 and 0.525 for women. The correlations show that although health outcomes are more similar the closer the reporting period, their absolute size suggests considerable mobility exists in GHQ scores over time. For example, all correlations off the lead diagonal are much smaller than 1 (1 indicating an absence of mobility) and less than one fifth are over 0.5. However, the non-zero correlation at the extremes suggests that this mobility operates around some underlying persistence in individual health trajectories.

More formal approaches to estimating the extent of mobility are achieved using two comparative measures. The first partitions unobserved variability in health status from an error components model into transitory and permanent components, and uses the proportion of total variability attributed to the permanent component as a measure of mobility. The following model is specified,

$$h_{it} = X'_{it}\beta + Z'_i\gamma + a_i + \varepsilon_{it}, i = 1, 2, \ldots, N; t = 1, 2 \ldots T_i$$

where h_{it} is the GHQ score for the *i-th* individual at time *t*. X_{it} represents a vector of time-varying explanatory variables and Z_i a vector of time-invariant explanatory variables, assumed to influence h_{it} but to be uncorrelated with the error term, $a_i + \varepsilon_{it}$. The total error is composed of a_i, an individual specific and time-invariant error and ε_{it}, the usual idiosyncratic error component. β and γ are conformably dimensioned vectors of parameters to be estimated. To allow for potential correlation between a_i and the set of time-varying regressors, X_{it}, the individual effect is parameterized to obtain a correlated random effects model (Mundlak 1978; Chamberlain 1984). The first estimate of mobility is based on the intra-unit correlation coefficient, ρ:

$$\rho = \frac{\sigma^2_a}{\sigma^2_a + \sigma^2_\varepsilon}$$

This coefficient represents the conditional correlation of GHQ scores across periods of observation. Should ρ be large, then individuals are said to experience relatively high persistence (low mobility) in health outcomes. Conversely, if the majority of unexplained variability is attributable to σ^2_ε, then individuals experience relatively high random fluctuations resulting in high mobility and low persistence in health outcomes. Estimates of ρ are calculated by maximum likelihood estimation.

A second measure of mobility is based on the estimated coefficient on lagged health status from a dynamic regression model. Here the set of regressors is augmented to include the previous period's GHQ score, in order to estimate the impact of previous health on current health. The general form of this dynamic model can be written as

$$h_{it} = \lambda h_{it-1} + X_{it}' \beta + Z_i' \gamma + v_{it}, \quad i = 1, 2, \ldots, N; \, t = 1, 2 \ldots T_i$$

where h_{it}, X_{it} and Z_i are defined as before. The model is estimated by ordinary least squares (OLS) (see Jarvis and Jenkins (1998) for an application to income mobility). A coefficient close to zero provides evidence of high mobility since current health is not a function of the previous period's health (conditional on X_{it} and Z_i). Accordingly, health outcomes fluctuate in a non-deterministic and random manner over time. Should the estimate of λ be positive and large, individuals are characterized by relatively low health mobility. A negative coefficient would indicate cyclical fluctuations in health outcomes over time.

Table 4.2 presents estimates of persistence for men and women. Gradients across the categories of the socioeconomic groups are clearly apparent. Less persistence is observed for ethnic groups other than white, for individuals with greater educational qualifications, for higher income groups, for younger individuals and for healthier individuals. Estimates derived from the lagged health variable estimated via OLS are larger than the mobility estimate derived from the proportion of variance attributable to the unobserved individual effect in the variance components model. In general, estimates of persistence for women are larger than those for men, but these differences are often negligible. The differences in estimates within the different socioeconomic groups are quite striking. For example, for men the increase in the estimated coefficient, $\hat{\rho}$, as one moves from degree or higher degree (DEGHDEG) to no qualifications (NOQUAL) is 50 per cent. The corresponding increase for the OLS coefficient, $\hat{\lambda}$, is 33 per cent. For women these differences are greater still at 78 per cent and 56 per cent respectively. Increases are even more pronounced across age quintiles so that the differences in estimates as one moves from the first (youngest) to the fifth (oldest) age quintile are men: 51 per cent for $\hat{\rho}$ and 68 per cent for $\hat{\lambda}$; women: 106 per cent and 78 per cent respectively. Estimates of mobility vary across social class groups with some indication of a gradient. For both men and women the lowest estimates, corresponding to greatest mobility, are observed for professional, managerial and technical and skilled non-manual workers. The highest coefficients (least mobility) are observed for the retired and other social class group.

Table 4.2 Mental health mobility across socioeconomic groups

	MEN		WOMEN	
	MLE $\hat{\rho}$	OLS $\hat{\lambda}$	MLE $\hat{\rho}$	OLS $\hat{\lambda}$
ALL DATA	.414 (.007)	.510 (.005)	.385 (.006)	.487 (.005)
ETHNICITY				
WHITE	.417 (.007)	.511 (.005)	.385 (.006)	.488 (.005)
OTHETH	.300 (.035)	.422 (.030)	.338 (.035)	.431 (.029)
EDUCATION				
DEGHDEG	.318 (.018)	.420 (.015)	.262 (.018)	.362 (.016)
HNDALEV	.379 (.013)	.483 (.010)	.314 (.014)	.425 (.011)
OCSE	.409 (.013)	.498 (.010)	.341 (.011)	.447 (.009)
NOQUAL	.469 (.012)	.557 (.009)	.466 (.010)	.564 (.007)
INCOME				
1st quintile	.477 (.015)	.567 (.011)	.436 (.014)	.519 (.011)
2nd quintile	.435 (.015)	.539 (.011)	.400 (.014)	.508 (.010)
3rd quintile	.386 (.016)	.453 (.012)	.397 (.014)	.494 (.010)
4th quintile	.367 (.015)	.472 (.012)	.327 (.013)	.439 (.011)
5th quintile	.329 (.015)	.451 (.012)	.295 (.013)	.417 (.011)
AGE				
1st quintile	.285 (.014)	.385 (.012)	.266 (.012)	.353 (.011)
2nd quintile	.354 (.015)	.456 (.012)	.316 (.014)	.425 (.011)
3rd quintile	.399 (.015)	.494 (.012)	.349 (.014)	.469 (.011)
4th quintile	.432 (.016)	.537 (.011)	.463 (.014)	.567 (.010)
5th quintile	.586 (.014)	.649 (.010)	.550 (.013)	.629 (.010)
SOCIAL CLASS				
PROF	.315 (.027)	.415 (.022)	.212 (.045)	.267 (.046)
MANTECH	.323 (.014)	.431 (.011)	.318 (.014)	.447 (.011)
SKNONM	.303 (.023)	.449 (.020)	.287 (.013)	.373 (.011)
SKMANAR	.376 (.014)	.464 (.011)	.375 (.030)	.450 (.023)
UNPSKL	.369 (.020)	.497 (.016)	.374 (.019)	.482 (.014)
UNEMP	.396 (.038)	.457 (.031)	.177 (.056)	.160 (.065)
FAMCARE	–	–	.398 (.105)	.497 (.012)
RETIRED	.585 (.014)	.651 (.010)	.522 (.012)	.629 (.009)
SCOTHER	.482 (.029)	.605 (.020)	.425 (.037)	.535 (.026)
HEALTH				
HEALTHY	.128 (.006)	.236 (.007)	.134 (.006)	.245 (.007)
UNHEALTHY	.208 (.009)	.348 (.009)	.160 (.007)	.305 (.008)

Source: Hauck and Rice (2003)
Notes:
1 Individuals are classified as being healthy if their mean GHQ score is lower than the sample mean GHQ score. Individuals are classified as being unhealthy if their mean GHQ score is higher than the sample mean GHQ score.
2 Too few observations for FAMCARE to provide reliable estimates for men.
3 MLE = Maximum likelihood estimator.

To summarize these findings, Hauck and Rice (2003) find evidence of substantial mobility in mental health. This is apparent for both men and women. Further, they find evidence of systematic differences in mobility across socioeconomic groups. In general, individuals from an ethnic origin other than white experience worse mental health outcomes (although these effects are not statistically significant) but greater mobility over time compared to white ethnic groups. Individuals from lower income groups are associated with greater mental ill-health but are also associated with greater persistence over time compared to individuals from higher income groups. Cross-sectional analyses find that mental health problems are concentrated among groups with low educational status (Henderson 1998). The results concur with this but also imply that mental health problems among low education groups are aggravated by the fact that they tend to be of a more permanent nature. Mental health deteriorates with age and becomes more permanent in nature. The unemployed, and individuals categorized as other social class, report worse GHQ scores than the baseline of skilled non-manual workers. Further, women occupied with family care report greater levels of mental illness compared to the baseline group. However, the retired and other social class group experience greatest persistence in outcomes over time.

The socioeconomic determinants of health

A recent paper by Contoyannis *et al.* (2004) explores the dynamics of SAH in the BHPS. The variable of interest is an ordered measure of SAH and, as for the GHQ score, the BHPS reveals evidence of considerable persistence in individuals' health status. So for example, men who report excellent health at wave 1 are most likely to report excellent health again at wave 2. If they change health status they are most likely to report good health. Those who report good health at wave 1 are most likely to report good health at wave 2 and if they change it is most likely to be to excellent health or fair health and the same pattern applies to all categories of SAH. Two possible sources of this persistence are unobservable heterogeneity – inherent individual differences in health that remain constant throughout the survey – and state dependence, such that an individual's previous experience of health influences their current health outcomes.

Econometric analysis of health based on longitudinal data needs to take account of the fact that the sample changes over time and, in particular, the results of the analysis may be influenced by attrition bias. Patterns of attrition in the BHPS data are illustrated in Table 4.3. This shows how the number of individuals among both men and women in the sample used by Contoyannis *et al.* evolves over the eight waves of the panel. The survival rate shows how the number of respondents declines so that, by the eighth wave, only 64 per cent of the original sample of men and 69 per cent of the original sample of women are included. The number of dropouts from the sample can be summarized by the attrition rate. This gives the number of individuals who drop out between two waves as a percentage of the number of respondents at the start of the period. This shows that the attrition rate is highest between waves 1 and 2 and 2 and 3 and then declines over time. So the overall attrition rate for men is 13 per cent between waves 1 and 2 and for women it is 12 per cent. What is striking about Table 4.3 is the evidence of health-related attrition. The final five columns show the attrition rates for those in different categories of SAH at the previous wave. Attrition rates are noticeably higher among those who report very poor health at the previous wave, providing evidence of health-related attrition, which may be a source of attrition bias in econometric models of health.

Contoyannis *et al.* (2004) develop an econometric model for self-assessed health (SAH). In the BHPS, SAH is an ordered categorical variable based on the question 'Please think back over the last 12 months about how your health has been. Compared to people of your own age, would you say that your health has on the whole been excellent/good/fair/poor/very poor?' As this is measured at each wave of the panel there are repeated measurements ($t = 1 \ldots T$) for a sample of individuals ($i = 1 \ldots n$):

$$h^*_{it} = \beta' x_{it} + \gamma' h_{it-1} + a_i + \varepsilon_{it} \; (i = 1, \ldots, N; \, t = 2 \ldots T_i)$$

This is modelled using a latent variable specification, which can be estimated using pooled ordered probit (with robust inference) and random effects ordered probit models. x includes measures of socio-economic status such as income and education. The presence of h_{it-1} is designed to capture state dependence and the influence of previous health history on current health. The error term is split into two components. The first captures time invariant individual hetero-geneity, while the second is the usual time varying idiosyncratic component. In this kind of application it is quite likely that the unobserved individual effect, which encompasses omitted variables that are not included in the survey, will be correlated with the other regressors, such as education and income. Also, it is well known that

Table 4.3 Sample size, dropouts and attrition rates by wave

Men

Wave	No. individuals	Full sample Survival rate	Dropouts	Attrition rate	Ex at t-1 Attrition rate	Good at t-1 Attrition rate	Fair at t-1 Attrition rate	Poor at t-1 Attrition rate	Vpoor at t-1 Attrition rate
1	4832								
2	4180	86.51%	652	13.49%	12.17%	13.45%	14.23%	14.63%	26.88%
3	3752	77.65%	428	10.24%	8.92%	9.51%	11.49%	14.58%	24.00%
4	3593	74.36%	159	4.24%	6.65%	7.40%	7.29%	8.52%	14.52%
5	3392	70.20%	201	5.59%	5.40%	7.42%	9.61%	9.72%	22.95%
6	3308	68.46%	84	2.48%	3.56%	3.05%	4.80%	12.16%	25.40%
7	3249	67.24%	59	1.78%	3.27%	4.46%	4.62%	9.65%	11.48%
8	3105	64.26%	144	4.43%	4.06%	4.43%	6.36%	7.00%	22.89%

Women

Wave	No. individuals	Full sample Survival rate	Dropouts	Attrition rate	Ex at t-1 Attrition rate	Good at t-1 Attrition rate	Fair at t-1 Attrition rate	Poor at t-1 Attrition rate	Vpoor at t-1 Attrition rate
1	5424								
2	4777	88.07%	647	11.93%	10.83%	11.81%	12.06%	13.16%	21.43%
3	4410	81.31%	367	7.68%	7.19%	6.94%	8.21%	11.33%	16.36%
4	4232	78.02%	178	4.04%	6.69%	5.82%	6.32%	11.53%	14.89%
5	4038	74.45%	194	4.58%	7.12%	5.15%	6.67%	8.61%	11.96%
6	3930	72.46%	108	2.67%	2.63%	3.40%	5.24%	9.27%	14.29%
7	3853	71.04%	77	1.96%	3.02%	3.34%	4.91%	8.26%	7.07%
8	3734	68.84%	119	3.09%	2.74%	3.32%	4.53%	5.16%	12.61%

Source: Contoyannis *et al.* (2004)

Table 4.4 Average partial effects on probability of reporting excellent health for selected variables

Men

	(1) Pooled model, balanced sample	(2) Pooled model, unbalanced sample	(3) Pooled model, IPW-1	(4) Pooled model, IPW-2	(5) Random effects, balanced sample	(6) Random effects, unbalanced sample
Ln(INCOME)	.009 (.004)	.009 (.004)	.009 (.004)	.011 (.005)	.013 (.006)	.012 (.005)
Mean Ln(INCOME)	.049 (.024)	.043 (.022)	.042 (.021)	.045 (.022)	.066 (.028)	.056 (.025)
DEGREE	.010 (.005)	.017 (.009)	.018 (.009)	.018 (.009)	.015 (.006)	.027 (.012)
HND/A	.019 (.009)	.021 (.011)	.021 (.010)	.022 (.011)	.028 (.011)	.030 (.013)
O/CSE	.016 (.008)	.020 (.010)	.020 (.010)	.020 (.010)	.024 (.010)	.028 (.012)
SAHEX(t–1)	.234 (.087)	.231 (.090)	.231 (.090)	.230 (.089)	.082 (.031)	.085 (.035)
SAHFAIR(t–1)	–.170 (.085)	–.163 (.084)	–.162 (.084)	–.162 (.083)	–.080 (.034)	–.077 (.036)
SAHPOOR(t–1)	–.242 (.167)	–.233 (.163)	–.232 (.162)	–.232 (.162)	–.151 (.077)	–.145 (.078)
SAHVPOOR(t–1)	–.260 (.198)	–.253 (.197)	–.255 (.199)	–.255 (.200)	–.184 (.104)	–.179 (.106)

Women

	(1) Pooled model, balanced sample	(2) Pooled model, unbalanced sample	(3) Pooled model, IPW-1	(4) Pooled model, IPW-2	(5) Random effects, balanced sample	(6) Random effects, unbalanced sample
Ln(INCOME)	.006 (.004)	.007 (.004)	.005 (.003)	.004 (.002)	.006 (.003)	.008 (.004)
Mean Ln(INCOME)	.028 (.016)	.025 (.015)	.029 (.017)	.030 (.017)	.039 (.020)	.033 (.018)
DEGREE	.037 (.020)	.034 (.019)	.036 (.020)	.039 (.022)	.049 (.024)	.044 (.022)
HND/A	.019 (.011)	.022 (.013)	.023 (.013)	.022 (.013)	.027 (.014)	.030 (.015)
O/CSE	.026 (.015)	.023 (.013)	.024 (.014)	.025 (.015)	.035 (.018)	.029 (.015)
SAHEX(t−1)	.220 (.095)	.206 (.092)	.205 (.091)	.208 (.092)	.082 (.038)	.074 (.035)
SAHFAIR(t−1)	−.132 (.078)	−.128 (.076)	−.127 (.075)	−.127 (.074)	−.064 (.034)	−.061 (.033)
SAHPOOR(t−1)	−.185 (.144)	−.182 (.142)	−.183 (.142)	−.183 (.142)	−.121 (.073)	−.118 (.072)
SAHVPOOR(t−1)	−.201 (.175)	−.198 (.173)	−.199 (.173)	−.199 (.173)	−.144 (.095)	−.144 (.097)

Source: Contoyannis et al. (2004)

in dynamic specifications the individual effect will be correlated with the lagged dependent variable. This gives rise to what is known as the *initial conditions problem*: that an individual's health at the start of the panel is not randomly distributed and will reflect the individual's previous experience and be influenced by the unobservable individual heterogeneity. To deal with the initial conditions an attractively simple approach suggested by Wooldridge (2002a) is used. This involves parameterizing the distribution of the individual effects as a linear function of initial health at the first wave of the panel and of the time means of the regressors, and assuming that it has a conditional normal distribution. As long as the correlation between the individual effect and initial health and the regressors is captured by this equation it will control for the problem of correlated effects. Its ease of implementation stems from the fact that a_i can be substituted back into the previous equation and the model can then be estimated as a pooled ordered probit or a random effects ordered probit using standard software to retrieve the parameters of interest.

Inverse probability weights are used to attempt to control for attrition (Woolridge 2002b). This works by estimating separate probit equations for whether or not an individual responds at each of the waves of the panel from 2 to 8. Then the inverse of the predicted probabilities of response from these models are used to weight the contributions to the log likelihood function in the pooled probit models for health. The rationale for this approach is that a type of individual who has a low probability of responding represents more individuals in the original sample and, therefore, should be given a higher weight. The appropriateness of this approach relies on the assumption that non-response is ignorable, conditional on the variables that are included in the probit models for non-response. If this assumption holds, then inverse probability estimates give consistent estimates with conservative inference, such that standard errors are overestimated.

Table 4.4 shows the average partial effects of selected variables on the probability of an individual reporting excellent health. These are given for pooled probit models with and without inverse probability weights and estimated on balanced and unbalanced samples and also for random effect specifications of the ordered probit models on balanced and unbalanced samples. The results show that state dependence is important: the estimated effects of lagged health status are large and highly statistically significant. What is more, a clear gradient is observed in the coefficients as they move from very poor to excellent previous health. So state dependence is one source of the observed persistence in SAH in the BHPS. Another source is individual heterogeneity: the intra-class correlation coefficient (ICC) shows the proportion of the overall variance of the error term which is attributable to the individual effect. Approximately 32 per cent of the latent error variance is accounted for by individual heterogeneity for both men and women.

There is little difference between the results and estimates of the pooled model with and without inverse probability weights. This suggests that while there is evidence of health-related attrition in the data, the average partial effects of socioeconomic variables and of lagged health status are not influenced by sample attrition. However, this does rely on the ignorability assumption built into the inverse probability weight approach and deserves further analysis.

Results for the income variables show that the effects of mean income are larger than those of current income and the effects of mean income are statistically significant, while those from current income are not. This deserves further investigation. The effect of mean income could be a genuine influence of permanent financial status on health or it could reflect the correlation between the unobserved individual effect and current income. For men, educational qualifications are positively associated with better health but we do not observe a clear gradient across individual qualifications. For women, educational qualifications are more significant and a clear gradient is observed.

To summarize these findings, there is clear evidence of health-related attrition in the BHPS data but it does not appear to distort estimates of our models for SAH. There is evidence of persistence in SAH and this is explained in part by state dependence, which is stronger among men than women, and by individual heterogeneity, with around 30–35 per cent of the unexplained variation accounted for by individual heterogeneity. There is evidence of a socioeconomic gradient by education and income with the long-run effect of income greater than the short-run effect.

CONCLUSIONS

The continuing concern over the level of inequalities in health has ensured that efforts to alleviate them have remained high on the policy agenda. Health economics has been at the forefront of developing analytic tools for the measurement and explanation of health inequalities and is well placed to continue to play a pivotal role in this important area. Methodological extensions to the literature on income inequality, together with the availability of high-quality longitudinal survey data, has extended the capacity of health economists to inquire into the nature and determinants of health inequalities. The availability of the ECHP has made detailed cross-country comparative analysis of health inequalities more amenable to empirical research, providing additional evidence on the extent of inequalities and how they are systematically related to socioeconomic factors in different health care systems.

An area that is under-researched, and that would benefit greatly from the input of health economists, is the evaluation of policy initiatives aimed at the reduction of inequalities in health. The proper evaluation of such initiatives is crucial if interventions are to be judged on the effectiveness (and cost-effectiveness) of their impact on the distribution of health. Economists have long been interested in the evaluation of social programmes, and to this end have developed a comprehensive toolkit of techniques upon which to draw (Blundell and Costa-Dias 2000). A combination of factors such as the non-experimental setting, identification of relevant risk groups, lags between intervention and outcome, and clear identification of the policy instrument all pose challenging issues for the analyst. The successful evaluation of policy initiatives aimed at the reduction in health inequalities should be afforded a prominent role in the future agenda on tackling inequalities in health.

ACKNOWLEDGEMENTS

Data from the British Household Panel Survey (BHPS) were supplied by the ESRC Data Archive. Neither the original collectors of the data nor the Archive bear any responsibility for the analysis or interpretations presented here. This chapter derives from the project 'The dynamics of income, health and inequality over the lifecycle' (known as the ECuity III Project), which is funded in part by the European Community's Quality of Life and Management of Living Resources programme (contract QLK6-CT-2002-02297). Nigel Rice is in part supported by the UK Department of Health programme of research at the CHE.

DISCUSSION
Matt Sutton

Jones and Rice present an important overview of the need for, and recent developments in, longitudinal econometric analysis of health inequalities. Given this focus, their review is inevitably a partial view of the contribution of economics to the study of health inequalities. The purpose of my discussion is to provide a broader backdrop and suggest some key challenges for future work.

The production of health is fundamental to health economics. All other components of health economics (such as the measurement and evaluation of health, evaluation of technologies, and health care market analysis) improve our understanding of how best to produce health. Even if viewed only as a positive exercise, the heterogeneity implicit in health inequalities can be used to understand the production function better. In normative terms, health is often seen as a fundamental good and inequalities in it are a priority for social action. The study of health inequalities should therefore attract economists, yet health determinants are a research focus for few (Maynard and Kanavos 2000).

Economists have contributed to inequalities research in a range of ways, providing commentary from a unique perspective on important policy documents (Maynard 1999), offering significant theoretical frameworks for analysing inequality and inequity (Mooney 1982; Culyer and Wagstaff 1993; Williams and Cookson 2000), and stylized (Evans and Stoddart 1990) and formal (Grossman 1972) economic models of health production. It is nevertheless surprising that the demand for health remains a relatively under-researched area (Grossman 2000), despite the existence of models highlighting the roles of education, risk aversion and health care consumption. Finally, economists have also contributed significantly to measurement, and below I give some strengths, weaknesses and priorities for the future in this area.

STRENGTHS

First, in tailoring measurement techniques from the study of income inequality, economists have added significantly to the health inequality analyst's toolbox. Although Mackenbach and Kunst (1997) concluded that there were deficiencies in the concentration index, many of their criticisms have been answered in more recent contributions in terms of significance testing (Kakwani *et al.* 1997), social weights (Wagstaff 2002) and interpretation (Koolman and van Doorslaer 2004).

Second, economists have been keen to retain the continuous nature of income in measuring health inequalities, rather than losing information through convenient but arbitrary banding. Third, health economists are keen to work with cardinal health outcomes (e.g. QALYs). Van Doorslaer and Jones' work on scaling ordinal health measures is a significant advance in avoiding analysis of dichotomized or ranked data (Koolman and van Doorslaer 2004). Recent developments in the decomposition of inequalities also provide useful insights. Health inequalities arise because income is correlated with health and because income is unequally distributed. Either or both of these factors can vary over time and between areas and suggest different policy responses.

There are other important economic contributions to measurement including the potentially biasing effects of two-stage standardization (Schokkaert and van de Voorde 2000; Gravelle 2003), analysis using non-linear models (Jones 2000) and comparisons of the effect of income measured in absolute terms or relative to reference groups (Wildman 2003).

WEAKNESSES

There are, however, some areas of weakness. While economists may be convinced that their inequality measures have desirable properties, more needs to be done to get them into the mainstream. Our thirst for ever more technical solutions also suggests a need for more attention to the details of data. It is notable that few studies offer precise details about the income variable used and are careful about which they select (Benzeval and Judge 2001). Although administrative data provide information on 100 per cent of individuals, they have been little used by economists for health inequality research. The challenges posed by its aggregate nature should in some senses be an attraction, and it offers very long-term trends and harder endpoints, such as mortality.

The quest to demonstrate new techniques tends to make us reach for what is available. The BHPS regularly contains only one health variable that can feasibly be treated as continuous – the 12-item GHQ. Health economists have generally been critical of researchers applying arbitrary scoring systems to health scales, yet the attraction of a 'continuous' health measure is, for some, hard to resist (Hauck and Rice 2003; Wildman 2003).

There has been recent criticism of a concentration on socio-economic inequality (Gakidou *et al.* 2000), which becomes more pointed with reference to economists' focus on income alone. Although it is possible to defend a socioeconomic focus, there are many possible dimensions of socioeconomic status and it will be important to continue to develop approaches that capture inequalities in a multiplicity of socioeconomic dimensions (Wagstaff and van Doorslaer 2004).

A final weakness of economic work in this area is the reporting of results. The techniques required are complex and there is no value in producing solutions that are 'simple but wrong'. What is required, however, is a more user-friendly front-end, such as that provided by the UK *Institute for Fiscal Studies* for communicating the consequences of income inequality to a non-specialist audience (Goodman and Shephard 2002). Such developments should not only include simple ways to present data and results, but also simulations of the consequences of changes in policy and the economy for average levels of health and the extent of health inequality.

SOME FUTURE PRIORITIES

I conclude with three broad recommendations for future work. First, that economic research on health inequalities should embrace a range of data sources, including longitudinal datasets where economists have been key to the design (such as the English Longitudinal Study of Ageing) and large-scale administrative datasets. Second, attention should be paid to the evaluation of policy initiatives (Benzeval *et al.* 2000) and to monitoring the effects of economic and policy changes and reporting them in accessible ways. Finally, in focusing on the determinants of health we should not forget the role of health services in determining health and the potential for inequities in access to health care services to contribute to socioeconomic inequalities in health.

REFERENCES

Acheson, D. (1998) *Independent Inquiry into Inequalities in Health*. London: HMSO.

Benzeval, M. and Judge, K. (2001) Income and health: the time dimension, *Social Science and Medicine*, 52: 1371–90.

Benzeval, M., Judge, K. and Taylor, J. (2000) Evidence on the relationship between low income and poor health: is the government doing enough? *Fiscal Studies*, 21(3): 375–99.

Blundell, R. and Costa-Dias, M. (2000) Evaluation methods for non-experimental data, *Fiscal Studies*, 21(4): 427–68.

Bommier, A. and Stechklov, G. (2002) Defining health inequality: why Rawls succeeds where social welfare theory fails, *Journal of Health Economics*, 21: 497–513.

Chamberlain, G. (1984) Panel data, in M. Intrilligator (ed.) *Handbook of Econometrics*, pp. 1247–318. Amsterdam: North-Holland.

Contoyannis, P., Jones, A.M. and Rice, N. (2004) The dynamics of health in the British Household Panel Survey (BHPS), *Journal of Applied Econometrics*, forthcoming.

Culyer, A. and Wagstaff, A. (1993) Equity and equality in health and health care, *Journal of Health Economics*, 12: 431–57.

Department of Health (2000) *The NHS Plan: A Plan for Investment, a Plan for Reform*. London: The Stationery Office.

Department of Health (2002) *Tackling Health Inequalities: Summary of the 2002 Cross-Cutting Review*. London: Department of Health.

Department of Health (2003) *Tackling Health Inequalities: A Programme for Action*. London: Department of Health.

Evans, R. and Stoddart, G. (1990) Producing health, consuming health care, *Social Science and Medicine*, 31(12): 1347–63.

Gakidou, E., Murray, C. and Frenk, J. (2000). Defining and measuring health inequality, *Bulletin of the World Health Organisation*, 78(1): 42–52.

Goodman, A. and Shephard, A. (2002) *Inequality and Living Standards in Great Britain: Some Facts*. Briefing Note No. 19. London: Institute for Fiscal Studies.

Gravelle, H. (2003) Measuring income related inequality in health: standardisation and the partial concentration index, *Health Economics*, 12(10): 803–19.

Grossman, M. (1972) On the concept of health capital and the demand for health, *Journal of Political Economy*, 80: 223–55.

Grossman, M. (2000) The human capital model, in J.P. Newhouse (ed.) *Handbook of Health Economics*. Amsterdam: Elsevier.

Hauck, K. and Rice, N. (2003) *A Longitudinal Analysis of Mental Health Mobility in Britain*. ECuity III Working Paper No. 9.

Henderson, C.E.A. (1998) Inequalities in mental health, *British Journal of Psychiatry*, 173: 105–9.

Jarvis, S. and Jenkins, S. (1998) How much income mobility is there in Britain? *The Economic Journal*, 108: 428–43.

Jones, A.M. (2000) Health econometrics, in J.P. Newhouse (ed.) *Handbook of Health Economics*. Amsterdam: Elsevier.

Jones, A.M. and López Nicolás, A. (2003) *Measurement and Explanation of Socioeconomic Inequality in Health with Longitudinal Data*. ECuity III Working Paper No.1.

Kakwani, N. (1980) *Income Inequality and Poverty. Methods of Estimation and Policy Implications*. Oxford: Oxford University Press.

Kakwani, N., Wagstaff, A. and van Doorslaer, E. (1997) Socioeconomic inequalities in health: measurement, computation and statistical inference, *Journal of Econometrics*, 77: 87–103.

Koolman, X. and van Doorslaer, E. (2004) *On the Interpretation of a Concentration Index of Inequality*. ECuity II Project Working Paper No. 4.

Le Grand, J. (1989) An international comparison of ages-at-death, in J. Fox (ed.) *Health Inequalities in European Countries*. Aldershot: Gower.

Lerman, R.I. and Yitzhaki, S. (1984) A note on the calculation and interpretation of the Gini index, *Economic Letters*, 15: 363–8.

Mackenbach, J.P. and Kunst, A.E. (1997) Measuring the magnitude of socioeconomic inequalities in health: an overview of available measures illustrated with two examples from Europe, *Social Science and Medicine*, 44(6): 757–71.

Maynard, A. (1999) Inequalities in health: an introductory editorial, *Health Economics*, 8(4): 281–2.

Maynard, A. and Kanavos, P. (2000) Health economics: an evolving paradigm, *Health Economics*, 9(3): 183–90.

Mooney, G. (1982) *Equity in Health Care: Confronting the Confusion*. Health Economics Research Unit Discussion Paper 11/82. Aberdeen: Aberdeen University.

Mundlak, Y. (1978) On the pooling of time series and cross-sectional data, *Econometrica*, 48: 69–85.

Murray, C.J.L. and Lopez, A.D. (1996) *The Global Burden of Disease*. Boston, MA: Harvard University Press.

Rao, V. (1969) Two decompositions of the concentration ratio, *Journal of the Royal Statistical Society*, Series A, 132: 418–25.

Schokkaert, E. and van de Voorde, C. (2000) *Risk Selection and the Specification of the Risk Adjustment Formula*. Centre for Economic Studies Discussion Paper, 2000/011. Leuven: University of Leuven.

Shorrocks, A. (1978) Income inequality and income mobility, *Journal of Economic Theory*, 19: 376–93.

van Doorslaer, E. and Jones, A.M. (2003) Inequalities in self-reported health: validation of a new approach to measurement, *Journal of Health Economics*, 22(1): 61–87.

van Doorslaer, E. and Koolman, X. (2002) *Explaining the Differences in Income-related Health Inequalities Across European Countries*. ECuity II Project Working Paper No.6.

van Doorslaer, E., Koolman, X. and Jones, A.M. (2003) *Explaining Income-related Inequalities in Doctor Utilisation in Europe*. ECuity II Project Working Paper No.5.

Wagstaff, A. (2002) Inequality aversion, health inequalities and health achievement, *Journal of Health Economics*, 21: 627–41.

Wagstaff, A. and van Doorslaer, E. (2000) Measuring and testing for inequity in the delivery of health care, *Journal of Human Resources*, 35(4): 716–33.

Wagstaff, A. and van Doorslaer, E. (2004) Overall versus socioeconomic health inequality: a measurement framework and two empirical illustrations, *Health Economics*, 13(3): 297–301.

Wagstaff, A., van Doorslaer, E. and Paci, P. (1989) Equity in the finance and delivery of health care: some tentative cross-country comparisons, *Oxford Review of Economic Policy*, 5: 89–112.

Wagstaff, A., Paci, P. and van Doorslaer, E. (1991) On the measurement of inequalities in health, *Social Science and Medicine*, 33: 545–57.

Wagstaff, A., van Doorslaer, E. and Watanabe, N. (2003) On decomposing the causes of health sector inequalities with an application to malnutrition inequalities in Vietnam, *Journal of Econometrics*, 112: 207–23.

Wanless, D. (2002) *Securing Our Future Health: Taking a Long-Term View*. Final Report. London: HM Treasury.

Wildman, J. (2003) Income related inequalities in mental health in Great Britain: analysing the causes of health inequality over time, *Journal of Health Economics*, 22(2): 295–312.

Williams, A. (1997) Intergenerational equity: an exploration of the 'fair innings' argument, *Health Economics*, 6: 117–32.

Williams, A. and Cookson, R. (2000) Equity in health, in J.P. Newhouse (ed.) *Handbook of Health Economics*. Amsterdam: Elsevier.

Woolridge, J. (2002a) *Simple Solutions to the Initial Conditions Problem in Dynamic, Nonlinear Panel Data Models with Unobserved Heterogeneity*. CEMMAP Working Paper CWP18/02. Centre for Microdata Methods and Practice, IFS and UCL.

Woolridge, J. (2002b) Inverse probability weighted M-estimators for sample stratification, attrition and stratification, *Portuguese Economic Journal*, 1: 117–39.

Yitzhaki, S. (1983) On the extension of the Gini index, *International Economic Review*, 24: 617–28.

5

REGULATING HEALTH CARE MARKETS

Richard Cookson, Maria Goddard and Hugh Gravelle

INTRODUCTION

Both the demand and the supply of health care are heavily regulated in all countries. The reasons are not hard to find. First, there are obvious externalities from infectious disease, although these are generally most significant in developing countries. Second, ill health is unpredictable at the individual level and can make a large difference to well-being, and health care is expensive. Hence individuals will wish to insure. But the existence of asymmetrical information, adverse selection and moral hazard make the operation of insurance markets problematic. Third, there are economies of organizing health care services at one site rather than dispersing it across locations. This, coupled with patient travel and distance costs, means that the production of health care is subject to a degree of local natural monopoly. Finally, unregulated market outcomes may be inequitable.

As a consequence, government intervention in most health care systems is extensive. In some cases this takes the form of tax financed compulsory public insurance, with zero prices for patients, and public ownership of providers, as in the UK National Health Service (NHS). Even in the USA the state is by far the largest provider of insurance and funder of care via Medicare and Medicaid and is a large producer of medical care via the Veterans Administration hospitals.

We focus, though not exclusively, on the regulation of providers and purchasers of secondary care, since this is the most expensive component of most health care systems. The markets for health care labour and particular inputs such as pharmaceuticals are left to other chapters. Our aim is to sketch out the policy questions, discuss their economic content, and give a brief overview of the relevant economic literature. We consider the implications for policy and for future research: what gaps are there in the theory and evidence base for policy?

The behaviour of provider and purchaser organizations depends on the incentives and constraints under which they operate. We organize our discussion under three headings:

- *Ownership*: who has what residual claims on the organization's assets and profits?
- *Contracts*: how do agreed rewards paid by one organization to another depend on actions and outcomes?
- *Market structure*: how do the number, size and location of organizations, and their ability to enter and exit the market, affect actions?

We define 'regulation' as the imposition of constraints on these characteristics of health care markets. The policy question is how to regulate ownership forms, contracts and market structure to improve performance.

The analysis is relevant to three general policy issues which we illustrate with examples from NHS secondary care. The first is *diversity in provider ownership* forms. Most health care systems are based on a mixed economy, incorporating both public and private ownership of assets. In England, most secondary care is currently supplied by NHS Trusts, which are public corporations, subject to borrowing constraints and to direction from the Department of Health (DoH). Over the next five years, they will be converted into Foundation Trusts. Foundation Trusts will have more freedom from central direction by the DoH but will still be subject to performance monitoring by the Healthcare Commission. They will also have to obtain a licence to operate from a separate regulator who can revoke their licence if they achieve very low ratings from the Healthcare Commission. They will be able to retain operating surpluses and the proceeds of asset disposals for investment purposes and will be allowed to develop 'spin-off' companies. They will also enjoy less restricted access to capital markets. However, their borrowing will count as part of the public sector borrowing requirement (PSBR) and they will not be able to pledge as security the assets they use to provide NHS services. Furthermore, they will be constrained to continue supplying services to the NHS, will not be able to take on more private practice and cannot be wound up or merged. In many countries, there is a trend towards providing some services outside the acute hospital setting, including short-stay inpatient services, daycase surgery and community based diagnostic and minor surgical procedures. In England, new types of providers called Treatment Centres (TCs) are being established to carry out such work. There will be 80 TCs by the end of 2005, 32 in the independent sector and the rest NHS-run, treating at least 250,000 patients a year.

Second, the *remuneration of providers* is often highly regulated in health care systems, and in England contracting arrangements will change with the introduction of cost per case payments for procedures, based on a centrally determined national price tariff (DoH 2002).

Third, *patient-driven competition* is a feature of many health care systems and in future in England patients are to be offered greater choice of provider. Currently 'Patient Choice' pilot schemes give patients a choice of provider for elective surgery after they have been waiting for six months. By the end of 2005, all patients requiring elective surgery are to be offered the choice of four or five providers at the point of referral from the general practitioner (GP).

OWNERSHIP

Ownership forms

There is a great variety of ownership forms in the production of health care, including the classic entrepreneurial firm, professional partnerships, quoted public companies, charities and public sector firms owned by local or central government. In no country is the 'for profit' private firm dominant: even in the USA in 1994 most hospitals (60 per cent) were run by private 'not for profit' firms and about 28 per cent were public (Sloan 2000). There are two key ownership questions. First, should providers be privately or publicly owned? Second, should providers and purchasers be vertically integrated, in the sense that the purchaser owns the productive assets and employs workers to produce care, or should purchasers make an agreement with the providers who own the assets and hire the workers?

Models of ownership

Public ownership of providers is only one of the regulatory mechanisms available to address the features of health care that make market provision and organization problematic. Although health care providers have a degree of local natural monopoly power, privately-owned providers can be subject to regulation. Consumption of care can be subsidized in response to the externalities arising from infectious diseases. The state can mitigate *ex ante* moral hazard by altering the relative prices of health-affecting activities (e.g. smoking, sport) through taxes and subsidies. Problems arising from adverse selection can be reduced by subsidizing the insurance of high-risk individuals. However, health care differs from many other commodities in the degree of information asymmetry regarding quality: providers are generally better informed than either the consumer or the purchaser about the patient's prognosis and the relative effectiveness of the treatment offered. Thus regulators may find it difficult to prevent for-profit firms from increasing profit by degrading quality, or offering unnecessary treatments, or cream-skimming low-risk patients.

There are also potential hold-up problems (Klein *et al.* 1978). The location of a hospital can affect both its production costs and the net value to patients of the care it produces. Hospital assets are long-lived and can be converted to other uses only at considerable cost. The hospital owner is thus vulnerable to exploitation by the purchaser once the asset is in place. Fear of such exploitation may lead the provider to choose inefficient locations or types of investment.

With complete long-term contracts the ownership of the assets is not important since the parties can provide appropriate incentives for investment by contracting. However, it may not be possible for the parties to write long-term contracts because it is difficult to specify all the possible contingencies in advance in ways which can be verified by third parties. The incomplete contract literature (Grossman and Hart 1986; Hart and Moore 1990; Hart 1995) examines the efficient choice of asset ownership when the parties cannot contract *ex ante* on cost-reducing or value-increasing investments because neither the actions nor their effects are observable by third parties. As a consequence, the split of the *ex post* gains from trade will be determined by bargaining after the investments have been made. Ownership of assets matters because it affects the default 'no agreement' payoffs of the parties. These determine relative bargaining power, the share of the gains from investment, and hence the incentives for making cost-reducing or quality-increasing investments.

The incomplete contracts framework has been applied to questions of public ownership. In Hart *et al.* (1997), the potential producer can make two costly types of investment: the first improves quality, while the second reduces the cost of production but also reduces quality. If the asset is privately owned, the producer will always reap the full rewards from cost-reducing investment but, because of incomplete contracting, only receives a proportion of the increased value from higher quality. Hence, under private ownership, the producer has too great an incentive for cost reduction and too small an incentive for investment in quality. If the asset is publicly owned, the producer is employed by the state and underinvests in both cost reduction and quality because of their weaker *ex post* bargaining power. Although the model was developed to consider the choice between private and public production, it is also relevant for the choice between having the public purchaser act as the producer, or having the public purchaser contract at arms length with a publicly-owned producer. The insight that whether the provider or the purchaser owns the asset affects their *ex post* bargaining power and hence their *ex ante* incentives is still valid.

Hart (2003) has also applied the framework to situations in which a public purchaser contracts with the private sector to build and run an asset. The question he addresses is whether the same private firm should build and manage the publicly-owned asset or whether the contracts should be 'unbundled' so that builder and manager are separate enterprises. He argues that if it is easier to specify the quality of building than the quality of service then the unbundled provision is likely to be better.

The incomplete contracts literature provides a useful framework but it seems some way from providing firm guidance on public versus private ownership of hospital assets and vertical integration of purchasers and providers. Hart (2003) stresses that his model is very preliminary and Hart *et al.* (1997) note that the analysis of health care requires a considerable generalization of their model. For example, costs and (to a lesser extent) some aspects of quality are partly measurable, and the range of contracts which can be written between provider and purchaser is consequently wider. De Meza and Lockwood (1998) point out that the market environment in which firms operate is crucial because it affects the options available in the event of bargaining breakdown and hence affects bargaining power and incentives.

Hart *et al.* (1997) briefly consider the possibility that public purchasers may not be benevolent social welfare maximizers. Shleifer (1998) argues that the possibility of corruption and of using public firms for patronage of favoured groups strengthens the case for private ownership. There is scope for further work along the lines suggested by the models in Tirole (2000) which attempt to marry the incomplete contracts approach with public choice models to design structures which provide appropriate incentives to purchasers and providers. With non-benevolent purchasers, separation of purchaser and provider may be more attractive because it makes it easier for third parties to evaluate the performance of both, since the contract may generate more information and the costs of value destroying political operation are more transparent.

The literature has also not yet addressed the issue that because assets have a long life the effects of investment decisions will persist after the relevant decision-makers have retired or moved on to other jobs. There will be inefficiency if selfish decision-makers care only about the effects that occur during their tenure and ignore sub-sequent effects: future returns from actions cannot be capitalized. This problem arises by definition in public organizations and in some types of private organization, such as workers' cooperatives.

Empirical evidence

Evidence from other industries does not support the plausible argument that costs will be lower in private firms than in public firms. Costs appear to be more greatly affected by the degree of competition than by ownership. For health care, Sloan (2000) concludes that the evidence (largely from the USA) does not suggest systematic differences in cost between for-profit and not-for-profit firms. There are, however, serious problems in controlling for quality and allowing for the costs of travel, distance and time that fall on patients. There is little firm evidence on the effects of ownership on quality of care.

In England, fundholding primary care practices can be regarded as an attempt to vary property rights by making practices bear more of the costs of their decisions to refer to secondary care. When budgets are held by health authorities or Primary Care Trusts, the financial effects of an additional referral by a practice are spread over all practices: incentives are attenuated. Dusheiko *et al.* (2003) showed that, in England, giving a general practice a budget equal to the cost of the elective care of their patients in the year before the practice became a fundholder led to a reduction in elective admissions. It also led them to 'play the system' by increasing their elective admissions in the year before fundholding (Croxson *et al.* 2001).

There is little evidence on the effect of the purchaser-provider split introduced in the NHS in 1991, in part because beforehand, under vertical integration, there was no pressure to produce some of the required data. To date no one has taken advantage of the fact that providers and purchasers have been reintegrated in Scotland but not in England.

PURCHASER-PROVIDER CONTRACTS

In this section we examine how the performance of provider organizations may be influenced by the incentives in purchaser-provider contracts. We focus on the cost, volume and quality of specific services, and do not examine the role of purchaser-provider contracts in achieving allocative efficiency (the most efficient mix of services) or equity (who gets what services).

Health care contracting

Contract theory distinguishes three main ways of remunerating providers. The first is a flat-rate payment, possibly conditional on a minimum volume of activity – this is known in the UK as a 'block contract'. The second is a piece-rate payment per unit of output – known as a 'cost per case contract' when the price is fixed, or a 'cost and volume contract' when the price varies according to the volume of output. The third is a cost-sharing payment involving partial reimbursement of reported costs. In the NHS, cost-sharing contracts are not common, although some implicit cost sharing may have occurred in 'sophisticated' block contracts which permit renegotiation if reported costs overrun anticipated costs (Chalkley and Malcomson 1998a).

A key feature of contracting for health care is that important aspects of quality of care are non-contractible. The purchaser has a multi-task agency problem (Holmstrom and Milgrom 1990). The purchaser wants the provider to perform multiple tasks (e.g. to deliver both quantity and quality of care) but poorer evidence is available on some of the tasks (quality) than others (volume). In these circumstances the optimal contract will give weaker, lower-powered incentives for quality than for volume. The agent thus faces an incentive to skimp on quality. One partial solution is to attempt to improve the indicators of quality by devising performance indicators. However, there will always remain aspects of performance that cannot be measured using management data (Smith 2002), so this just restates the purchaser's problem as: how to raise quality above the minimum level enforceable through performance management?

One obvious economic mechanism for raising quality is competition between providers driven by patient demand. If patients have choice of provider, and are fully informed about quality, then competition between providers to attract patients can serve to raise quality. Under these circumstances, cost per case contracts will be optimal (Chalkley and Malcomson 1998b). However, patients may have limited scope for choice, and patient perceptions of quality may be imperfect. If so, the optimal contract depends on the degree to which providers have non-monetary objectives concerning quality of care. A block contract will only be optimal in the unlikely case that the provider is fully benevolent (i.e. cares as much about patient welfare and as little about its own income as the purchaser). A pure cost per case contract is unlikely to be efficient when providers are not fully benevolent, because payments designed to induce an efficient activity level will yield incentives for skimping on quality (Chalkley and Malcomson 1998a). A cost-sharing contract, by contrast, may give incentives to over-provide quality, so long as providers care to some extent about quality, which may help explain the high costs of the US Medicare system prior to 1983 (Weisbrod 1991). If providers are partly benevolent, therefore, the optimal contract may involve partial retrospective cost sharing combined with a cost per case payment (Ellis and McGuire 1990). The role of cost sharing here is to induce partly benevolent providers to raise quality of care above the minimum contractible level, by partially reimbursing the extra costs of higher quality.

Providers may also be able to reduce costs, without reducing quality, by more efficient use of inputs. The contracting literature assumes that cost-reducing effort is non-contractible and that providers face the non-monetary costs of making such effort. The problem is: how can the purchaser ensure that providers take appropriate steps to improve efficiency, when it is impossible to specify in advance exactly what these steps are? Cost sharing will dilute the incentive to engage in cost-reducing effort, so it will only be possible to attain either efficient quality, or efficient cost-reducing effort, but not both (Chalkley and Malcomson 1998a).

If the problem of quality skimping can be dealt with by policy

instruments other than contracting (such as performance management, or patient choice), then cost per case contracts may be
an attractive way of attaining efficient cost-reducing effort while
increasing activity rates. One approach is 'yardstick competition'
(Shleifer 1998). This sets a price per case, equal to the average of the
marginal costs of all other providers, plus a flat-rate 'break even'
payment. Like the Medicare prospective payment system (PPS) in
the USA, the NHS financial flows reforms of 2002 can be viewed as a
practical approximation to yardstick competition. The idea is to give
high marginal cost providers an incentive to engage in cost-reducing
effort, while preserving the incentive of low marginal cost providers
to increase activity levels. However, closing down inefficient providers
may be problematic in some health care systems.

In keeping with the existing health contracts literature, we have
focused on the problem of incentives for providers to under-perform
on non-contractible aspects of performance – a hidden action problem. However, there is also a problem of hidden information. Providers will know more about the illness severity of individual
patients than the purchaser. Price adjustments for severity and case-
mix built into Healthcare Resource Groups (HRGs) are inevitably
imperfect. This gives providers an incentive to treat only low-risk
patients whose expected cost of treatment is below the standard
HRG price (Newhouse 1983). This can be done either through
'cream-skimming' (e.g. tailoring facilities to attract low-risk patients)
or 'patient-dumping' (e.g. wrongly claiming that the hospital does
not have facilities to treat high-risk patients) (Folland *et al.* 2001).

Empirical evidence

Most of the evidence on the effects of contract design in health care
comes from the introduction of the PPS to US Medicare in 1983.
PPS was a major shift from cost-sharing to cost per case contracts,
with most payments based on the patient's diagnosis related group.
Theory predicts that this shift should reduce both costs and quality,
through a combination of quality skimping and increased cost-
reducing effort. Although it is always hard to pinpoint the precise
cost of particular services, given that hospitals are multi-product
firms, there is considerable evidence that PPS did indeed reduce costs
[from studies of length of stay and other service-specific resource
inputs] (summarized in Chalkley and Malcomson 2000). Evidence
that quality was reduced is less clear-cut. Studies using readily available quality data such as readmission rates and mortality rates tend

to find no overall effect (Cutler 1995). However, such measures are inevitably crude. The fall in treatment numbers following the introduction of PPS (Hodgkin and McGuire 1994) may be indirect evidence that some aspects of quality worsened: part of the explanation may be that patient demand responded to lower quality. The finding of Ellis and McGuire (1996) that 40 per cent of the observed reduction in psychiatric length of stay may be attributed to quality-skimping reductions in treatment intensity as opposed to changes in practice style, also suggests a quality reduction.

There is clearly scope for further econometric research in this area using data from the many other countries that have experimented with fixed price payments – not least the fixed price HRG reforms in England.

Incentives and objectives

Standard models of purchaser-provider contracts assume that the degree of provider benevolence is unaffected by the type of contract. However, the introduction of stark financial incentives and/or intrusive performance management regimes may reduce or eliminate benevolent motivation. The consequent loss of professional autonomy may alter the behaviour of consultants and other key medical staff from that of public-spirited 'knights' to self-interested 'knaves' (Le Grand 1997; Brennan and Hamlin 2000). In the behavioural economics literature, this phenomenon is known as 'motivational crowding out' of intrinsic benevolent motivations by extrinsic financial motivations (Frey 1997).

Brennan (1996) has also argued that institutional design should take account of the heterogeneity of individual preferences. Different types of contract containing different mixes of income and non-pecuniary rewards will attract different types of worker. Thus the type of contract which may be optimal for doctors may differ from that which is optimal for nurses, for cleaners, porters and accountants. The greater the scope of information asymmetry the more likely it is that the optimal contract will place relatively less weight on income and more on other job characteristics which are more likely to appeal to individuals with greater degrees of altruism.

Missing models?

Research in health economics has tended to proceed on the assumption that regulators are essentially benevolent in the sense that they pursue policy objectives relating to the good of society as a whole. By contrast, public choice theory assumes that the behaviour of government agencies is best understood in terms of the selfish personal and political interests of government officials (Mueller 2003). There is clearly scope for developing public choice models of the contracting process to analyse the behaviour of non-benevolent purchasers, and of multiple national and local purchasers with overlapping jurisdictions and potentially conflicting objectives.

There is also scope for research to apply dynamic models of long-term relationships to NHS contracting, including issues of reputation in maintaining quality of care and issues of commitment in making long-term investments (Chalkley and Malcomson 2000). Hospital assets are long-lived, and the dynamics of long-term relationships in health care merit explicit analysis in models of the contracting process. Such models may also need to incorporate ownership incentives, since these will affect the gains to investment in reputation.

MARKET STRUCTURE

The existence of a concentrated market and the exercise of market power in the interests of providers rather than consumers can produce a welfare loss (Cowling and Mueller 1978). Alternatively, the nature of the cost structure may be such that monopoly may be the most efficient mode of provision, exploiting the existence of economies of scale or scope and passing on reduced costs in the form of lower prices.

Concentration, price, cost and quality

Empirical evidence

Most empirical work in the health care sector has investigated the relationship between market concentration on the supplyside – as a proxy for market power – and costs/prices. Much of the evidence comes from the USA hospital sector where anti-trust policy has focused on the potential anti-competitive effects of mergers. In the USA there is a trend towards consolidation, with many smaller areas dominated by a single hospital and even larger urban areas having just two or three main providers (Arnould *et al.* 1997; Gaynor and Haas-Wilson 1999). Studies (from the USA and UK) of mergers have generally found evidence of only modest cost savings unless one of the merging hospitals closes (for summaries see Goddard and Ferguson 1997; Capps *et al.* 2002; Fulop *et al.* 2002) or capacity is substantially reduced in other ways (Dranove and Lindrooth 2003).

The main conclusion arising from US empirical studies is that there is a positive association between increased concentration and price (see the summaries by Dranove and White 1994; Goddard and Ferguson 1997; Capps *et al.* 2002; Abraham *et al.* 2003), though there is some debate about whether this holds only in the case of for-profit hospitals (Lynk 1995; Dranove and Ludwick 1999; Keeler *et al.* 1999; Lynk and Neumann 1999). Health care providers often set prices and quality simultaneously so research has also investigated the quality concentration link (using various measures of quality, including mortality and range of services offered) but the evidence is mixed and no definitive conclusions can be drawn (Ho and Hamilton 2000; Sari 2002; Volpp *et al.* 2003).

UK research has focused on policies that seek to stimulate supply-side competition (e.g. the 'internal market' 1991–7), rather than studying mergers directly. Although greater competition appears to be linked with lower prices (Propper and Soderlund 1998), evidence on concentration-cost relationships is limited and results mixed. Greater competition was found to be associated with poorer quality as measured by 30-day in-hospital death rates following emergency admission for acute myocardial infarction (Propper *et al.* 2002a, 2002b).

Measuring competition

A crucial issue is how markets are defined. Empirical studies in health care have almost always used geographical rather than product-based definitions. US studies have tended to define markets using administrative boundaries, whereas in the UK most research has either looked at patient flow data (based on the 'shipments' approach to markets) or has used simple rules-based definitions (e.g. counting providers per population within a certain travel time). Capps *et al.* (2002) have recently proposed defining markets in terms of the group of providers who could implement a small but significant non-transitory increase in price (SSNIP). The methods chosen to define markets can have a substantial impact on the results of analysis (Silvia and Leibenlutt 1998) and there has been little theoretical work undertaken on justification for particular approaches.

Economies of scale

The literature on scale economies in hospitals is extensive (mainly from the USA and UK) and has produced mixed results (Cowing *et al.* 1983; Aletrez *et al.* 1997; Gaynor and Vogt 2000; Posnett 2001). Some of the variation is accounted for by differences in methodology. The techniques used include regression studies of hospital cost and production functions, data envelopment analysis (to identify minimum efficient scale) and survival analysis (based on the assumption that hospitals that are too small or too large will lose market share to those at optimum size). Posnett (2001) documents some of the methodological issues arising and concludes that where economies of scale *are* found, they appear to be exploited at the level of 100–200 beds and diseconomies do not arise until around 300–600 beds.

There is also a large literature exploring the link between activity volume and quality, but again with mixed results and methodological shortcomings such as failure to control adequately for case mix. A systematic review by Sowden *et al.* (1997) concluded that in the few specialities where a positive association remains after adjustment for case-mix, the effects are at relatively low levels of activity and are unlikely to be relevant given current clinical practice. However, a more recent systematic review, including later studies, concluded that there was evidence of a volume-outcome link at both physician and hospital levels (Gandjour *et al.* 2003).

This research does not identify the causes of volume-quality relationships, but has provoked fierce debate about the policy implications that can be drawn for small hospitals and physicians working at low volumes of activity (Luft 2003; Sheikh 2003a, 2003b).

Purchaser size

The influence of market structure on the demand side must also be considered. The exercise of monopsony power can reduce provider profits and, in some circumstances, consumer welfare. In the USA, empirical work has focused on potential monopsony power in the health insurance market, especially in the light of the growth of managed care. As Gaynor and Vogt (2000) point out, most analyses suggest a negative relationship between purchaser market share and prices. In the UK, there is some evidence to suggest that purchasers with larger market shares (district health authorities) obtained lower prices from hospitals (for certain procedures) compared with the much smaller GP fundholders (Propper and Soderlund 1998).

Small numbers

Bi-lateral or multi-lateral bargaining is a feature of many health care markets (Pauly 1998). While bilateral monopoly can produce efficient outcomes in certain situations, the conditions required are restrictive (Chalkley and Malcomson 1998a). In other cases there are no general welfare results and much depends on the relative bargaining power of agents and the relative elasticity of demand and supply in the markets. Measuring bargaining power is not straightforward and little empirical work has been undertaken. Brooks *et al.* (1997) provide an interesting exception, using Nash bargaining model to structure an empirical analysis of bargaining between insurers and hospitals, in which they find that hospitals have greater bargaining power.

Entry and exit

Empirical evidence

Even relatively concentrated markets can be competitive if there is a credible threat of entry by new providers. Entry barriers can be exogenous (e.g. economies of scale, government licensing) and/or endogenous in that existing providers may deter new entry (e.g. limit pricing).

Much of the empirical work on the existence of entry barriers in health care markets has focused on physicians and networks in the USA and also on health maintenance organizations (HMOs) (Newhouse *et al.* 1982; Feldman *et al.* 1993; Feldman and Given 1998; Haas-Wilson and Gaynor 1998). A recent study of the impact of entry on the quantity of services supplied concludes that entry stimulated significantly greater competition, especially when a new hospital entered a single-hospital market, but subsequent entry had a lesser effect (Abraham *et al.* 2003).

Models

Models of entry and exit have been applied to longitudinal data on HMO entry and exit in the USA (summarized by Abraham *et al.* 2003). It would be possible to adapt these for use elsewhere, in order to establish the impact on entry and exit of: characteristics of the product and geographical markets; characteristics of the providers that enter and exit; and the nature of the regulatory regime. Similarly, entry into markets for coronary artery bypass graft (CABG) surgery has been examined in the USA (Chernew *et al.* 2002). Dafny (2003) used a model of entry deterrence to examine how far incumbents exploit the potential link between surgical volume and quality by manipulating volumes so as to create barriers to entry.

Of particular interest is the approach taken to exit when governments have an interest in supporting or bailing out providers who would otherwise fail to survive. Kornai *et al.* (2003) review a range of economic models explaining the behaviour of organizations that face soft, rather than hard, budget constraints, due to their expectation that a 'supporting' organization (usually the government) will intervene if they face financial failure, rather than allowing them to exit the market. They document the circumstances under which providers may be less efficient when they perceive their budget constraint to be soft. This approach is relevant to health care organizations, regardless of whether they are privately or publicly owned, and Kornai *et al.* document several possible motivations for bailing out such organizations, including the protection of prior investments, paternalism, enhancement of political popularity and protection of the reputation of those at the top of the hierarchy. The impact on the behaviour of organizations that expect to be rescued, rather than allowed to exit, has been the subject of empirical research in many non-health care sectors and a similar approach would be very relevant in the UK where exit (at least of entire hospitals) is usually prevented by government intervention.

POLICY IMPLICATIONS

What does the literature imply for regulatory policy?

In many health care systems where public funding or provision dominates, attempts have been made to sharpen the incentives faced by purchasers and providers (e.g. New Zealand, the Netherlands). In the UK, the imposition of uniform fixed prices for care via the Flow of Funds reforms is intended to give providers an incentive to reduce costs. The incentives will be increased by the ability of public providers to retain surpluses for investment. The effect on quality will depend on the degree of provider altruism and on the ability of purchasers to observe quality and to switch between providers.

The NHS has also started to adopt the sort of competitive mechanisms used in other countries: (i) payer-driven competition (PCTs switching contracts) and (ii) patient-driven competition (patients exercising choice of provider and funding following the patient). The success of this policy change will depend on the ability to develop better indicators of quality. Competition can only enhance quality of care if purchasers are well-informed about quality. In addition, it is not clear how far Primary Care Trusts are willing or able to act as aggressive purchasers (Baxter, Le Grand & Weiss 2003). The evidence on the effect of purchaser size suggests that smaller purchasers have less bargaining power, so the replacement of 100 health authorities by 304 PCTs may have reduced the bargaining power of purchasers.

Forcing purchasers to offer choice to patients may, if patients take up the choices, extend the market geographically and enhance competition. The relevant markets will be determined by patient willingness to travel, perceptions of quality and availability of information. As providers are to be price-takers, investigating the impact of enhanced competition will not be straightforward, requiring an analysis of cost and quality, rather than price data.

The NHS financial reforms may also have implications for equity, in particular geographical and socioeconomic equity of access to elective care. The imposition of a national tariff means that purchasers who currently deal with low-cost providers will find that their budget buys less care for their patients. There may also be exacerbation of inequalities in access if lower socioeconomic groups face greater barriers to exercising their new choice options.

Entry into UK health markets is heavily regulated by licensing requirements for the medical profession; by quality standards set by government and the professions (e.g. Royal Colleges) that limit new entry (e.g. minimum volume requirements); by control of location of GPs (until 2001) by the Medical Practices Commission; and by strict central control of new developments requiring major public capital investment. In the UK, new entry often takes the form of existing providers expanding into new service areas. At present this is controlled mainly through the purchaser-provider contractual relationship, mediated by involvement from other bodies such as the strategic health authorities. There are also some examples of regulation aimed at enhancing, rather than limiting, entry – for example, the Office of Fair Trading proposals to abolish pharmacy control of entry.

The impact on the UK health care market will depend on the entry conditions to be decided by the government – for example, the commitment made to private providers, the prices they are to be paid and their ability to attract sufficient labour. Often, entry regulation is 'captured' by incumbents. Recent cross-country research has linked heavy regulation of entry to higher levels of corruption and larger unofficial economies, rather than better-quality goods (Djankov *et al.* 2001). However, in England entry conditions appear to be designed in favour of the new entrants – for example, independent treatment centres (TCs) are to have access to NHS labour (albeit on a temporary basis) and there are examples where NHS TCs have been able to sign only very short-term contracts (12 months) with Primary Care Trusts in order to facilitate patient choice, whereas the independent TCs have five-year contracts. The health minister recently claimed that entry conditions will be used to 'disturb the old comfortable pattern in the NHS' (*Health Services Journal* 2003).

In many markets entry can lead to exit, as some providers fail to compete. In the UK, there is concern that transferring part of the core business outside the acute hospital will threaten the financial viability of some NHS hospitals. Traditional providers of private care may also find themselves out of business if TCs are able to undercut them in both waiting time and price. Past policy has been to prevent purchasers transferring major portions of their business from their local NHS providers, though mainly because of the perceived political cost rather than because of any assessment of the effects on the total costs and benefits of alternative service configurations. But, without an exit policy, measures to encourage entry will fail to achieve their potential to reduce costs and improve quality. Moreover, exit policies have to be convincing if they are to have an impact on the behaviour of providers and, as Kornai *et al.* (2003) suggest, this requires regulators to *demonstrate* their commitment to enforcing the policy rather than merely asserting it.

IMPLICATIONS FOR RESEARCH

We noted the potential areas for developments in the literature concerned with ownership, contracts and market structure in earlier sections, so we conclude by highlighting three general areas of theoretical development that require attention: public choice models, provider preferences and asymmetrical information.

Public choice models

Most formal health economics policy analysis follows the traditional normative welfare economics framework in which a benevolent social decision-maker pursues social welfare objectives, subject to resource and informational constraints. It ignores the political realities of health care decision-making, treating political factors as unfortunate constraints on the optimal decision. There has been very little health economic analysis in the public choice tradition with explicit positive models of incompletely altruistic regulators and purchasers as rational actors in the political market-place.

A public choice, rather than public interest, perspective would suggest less focus on regulation as a means of protecting the consumer and more on who gains from regulation and why there is potential for regulatory failure (Stigler 1971). Regulation may be captured not only by the incumbents but by a range of different interest groups (or the regulator itself), depending on the negotiation, bargaining and rent-seeking activities of these groups (Peltzman 1989; Laffont and Tirole 1991). Although much of the relevant economic theory has been developed within the context of government regulation of the private sector, the principles can also be applied to government regulation of public bodies (James 2000; Ashworth *et al.* 2002; Guerin 2003).

Many countries have witnessed an expansion in regulatory control in health care. In the UK there has been growth in regulation in some areas (Shaw 2001; Walshe 2002), alongside deregulation in other areas (e.g. Foundation Hospitals). These apparently contradictory developments may have been driven by the interests of particular groups. Related to this is the under-researched issue of *who* should regulate health care markets (Propper 1995a, 1995b). Proliferation of regulators with different, and often conflicting, responsibilities can create adverse effects. A recent analysis focused on a situation where two hierarchical levels of regulation co-existed with overlapping jurisdictions. It found that the possibility of intervention by the higher tier may 'crowd out' information acquisition by the lower tier, increasing the chances that the lower tier regulator is captured by providers (Bentz 2001). Failure to coordinate government regulation of physician services can lead to the sort of suboptimal outcomes (e.g. excessive costs and over-provision of care) that the regulation was meant to address (Rizzo and Sindelar 1996).

Provider preferences

A distinguishing feature of health economics is the willingness to consider models in which *providers* do not always have selfish preferences. This has typically taken the form of adding an additional argument to the objective function of providers to reflect a concern for patients. But the possibility that preferences are in part determined by the power of incentives and ownership structures has received little attention. Since providers are typically large and complex organizations whose members are unlikely to share the same preferences it would also be worthwhile considering how to model decision-making in provider organizations. By opening the black box we may gain some insight into the circumstances in which it is safe to model them as acting as if they had a well-behaved utility function.

Asymmetrical information

Asymmetry of information between providers, patients, purchasers and regulators is crucial to much of the modelling of behaviour and the derivation of optimal regulatory policies. Little attention has been paid to how decision-makers can improve their information, the incentives for doing so, and implications for behaviour. For example, the advent of information gathering and producing organizations like the Healthcare Commission and Dr Foster, the introduction of the electronic patient record, the linking of routine databases, and the reduction in the costs of acquiring information via the web, may reduce problems arising from asymmetry.

CONCLUSIONS

Assessment of alternative policies requires empirical analysis. Even well-developed, positive models will typically provide only qualitative guidance about the effects of policy parameters. The choice between policies will require information on the magnitude of effects, not just their sign. Much of the empirical evidence cited in this chapter derives from the USA, where the financial and administrative processes are such that good datasets are generally available. In the UK, health care datasets are improving in coverage and quality, though there have been some retrograde steps under the rubric of 'light touch' regulation. For example, we know a lot less about the activities of the 30 per cent of general practices that now have Primary Medical Service (PMS) contracts than those on General Medical Service (GMS) contracts because one of the inducements to practices to adopt PMS was a reduction in 'form filling'. The new GMS GP contract will generate a large amount of data on GP quality-related activities but it is not yet clear that it will be centrally collated, though it will have to be collected locally in order to pay practices. Hospital activity data quality and coverage is improving but there is still some way to go. For example, research on the patterns of use is hampered by the fact that with multiple-site Trusts it is not possible accurately to identify the site where treatment takes place.

New policies are typically introduced in a way that makes evaluation difficult. With a once-for-all national implementation the best one can do is a before and after study, often with inadequate data on the 'before'. It would be possible in many cases to phase in the implementation of policies across areas so that 'natural' experiments provide some scope for identifying the effects of policy and, hence, improving it.

DISCUSSION
Brian Ferguson

The chapter contains an excellent discussion of the issues concerning the regulation of health care markets. The authors clearly and comprehensively set out regulatory issues under three headings: ownership forms, contractual relationships and market structure. They focus largely on the market for hospital care.

Although much of the discussion is generalizable beyond a UK context, there are three important policy developments specific to the NHS. The first is a re-visiting of the concept of self-governing hospital trusts (Secretaries of State for Health 1989), now labelled 'Foundation Trusts'. These will, in theory, have defined capital and labour market freedoms and the ability to retain operating surpluses (more later). The recent *Reforming NHS Financial Flows* guidance (DoH 2002) is the second key policy development. This essentially signals a move towards cost-per-case payments for specific procedures, based upon a centrally determined national price tariff. Third, the Patient Choice initiative emphasizes the government's focus upon access to services: patients are to be given a choice of provider after waiting more than six months for elective surgery, with a target by the end of 2005 that patients will be offered a choice of four or five providers at the point of referral (DoH 2001).

The economic rationale underpinning these developments is simplistic, and comprises three elements. First, hospital providers are to be given incentives to be 'profitable'. Second, price uncertainty and the impact of artificial variations in cost among providers are to be minimized through the use of national price tariffs. Partly through this, and partly through the Patient Choice initiative, the aim is to stimulate activity and reduce costs. In passing, it should be noted that there is an inherent tension across these disparate initiatives: on the one hand there is an attempt to reduce variations in costs among hospital providers; on the other hand there is the scope – through the proposed labour market freedoms – to increase variation in local costs. Such variation may well be 'artificial' unless one believes that all wage rates truly reflect marginal rates of return in the NHS.

The authors recognize and explain one of the inherent pitfalls in these proposals: namely the existence of asymmetric information. The whole subject of measuring quality deserves further attention (more later) but is an obvious area of interest for whoever is regulating health care. To this may be added the obvious maxim that competition requires winners and losers: the internal market of the 1990s did not lead to 'inefficient' hospitals going out of business, and nor will this set of reforms. To what extent will hospitals be allowed, in practice, to retain surpluses in what remains a largely cash-limited system?

One important implication of asymmetric information and incomplete contracts is that regulators may find it difficult to prevent providers from degrading quality in order to increase profit. In the case of publicly-owned assets, there may be under-investment in both cost reduction and quality improvement. Consideration needs to be given to situations where the commissioner of services is also the provider, an important development since the creation of Primary Care Trusts. The concept of Primary Care Trusts as benevolent social welfare maximizers (if indeed they are) sits somewhat uncomfortably alongside proposed incentives to profit-maximize as providers.

The purchaser's problem may be stated as how to raise quality above the minimum level enforceable by centralized performance management. Cost-per-case contracts may be optimal if quality is fully observable and real patient choice exists, but to what extent, in practice, will competition be driven by well-informed patient demand? Providers may be able to reduce costs without reducing quality through more efficient use of inputs, but this implies the scope to close down 'uneconomic' departments. It also assumes that clinical and managerial objectives are aligned, whereas in practice there is a complex set of agency relationships in the provision of hospital care.

There are some important 'macro' questions such as who should ideally regulate health care markets. The authors point to the scope of public choice models to inform this debate, focusing on issues such as who stands to gain from regulation and why there is potential for regulatory failure. It is important to recognize the complexity of the current system, with multiple regulators at different geographical levels. For example, how are the activities and roles of strategic health authorities, the Healthcare Commission and local authorities (through health scrutiny) to be defined and reconciled?

There are several policy implications. First, the success of *Reforming NHS Financial Flows* (DoH 2002) will depend critically on the ability of public providers to retain surpluses for investment. Second, purchasers need to be able to observe quality, and better indicators of quality are needed to facilitate this. Third, Primary Care Trusts need to be both willing and able to encourage real patient choice. Fourth, there are important equity implications to be assessed and monitored over time – potentially through diverting funds away from high-cost hospitals towards more 'efficient' ones, and also potentially exacerbating socio-economic variations through choice being exercised by different groups of patients and carers. Finally, if serious consideration is not given to an 'exit policy', measures to encourage market entry will fail to achieve their full potential to reduce costs and enhance quality.

What strategies exist for taking forward research in this complex area? The two extremes are to throw up hands in horror and say 'it's all too difficult', or to 'return to the back room' and espouse the need for well-designed randomized controlled trials. Neither of these has much appeal. The middle ground is to continue to identify and model incentives and constraints in the system, and to assess the welfare implications of alternative policies through sound empirical analysis.

As a footnote to this debate on regulation, it is suggested that the quality and outcomes framework proposed under the new GMS contract (DoH 2003) offers an opportunity to explore many of the issues contained in the chapter from both a methodological and empirical perspective. The proposals in the new GMS contract have at their core the notion that income will (partly) be determined by measurable aspects of quality, and that there will be explicit financial incentives to reach higher levels of quality. The concept of 'aspiring' to a particular level of quality resonates with the central commissioning problem stated earlier: how to raise quality above the minimum level. The proposed framework does not, of course, overcome the complex problems of defining and measuring quality, and there remain some unanswered questions about how the system will 'minimize bureaucracy' in practice (there is surely scope for significant increases in transaction costs). Nevertheless, it is tentatively suggested that primary care may offer a rich testing ground for many of the regulatory issues raised in this chapter.

REFERENCES

Abraham, J., Gaynor, M. and Vogt, W. (2003) *Entry and Competition in Local Hospital Markets*, CMPO Working Paper 03/088, University of Bristol.

Aletrez, V., Jones, A. and Sheldon, T. (1997) Economies of scale and scope, in J. Posnett (ed.) *Concentration and Choice in Health Care*. London: RSM Press.

Arnould, R.J., DeBrock, L.M. and Radach, H.L. (1997) The nature and consequences of provider consolidations in the US, in J. Posnett (ed.) *Concentration and Choice in Healthcare*. London: RSM Press.

Ashworth, R., Boyne, G. and Walker, R. (2002) Regulatory problems in the public sector: theories and cases, *Policy and Politics*, 30(2): 195–211.

Baxter, K., Le Grand, J. and Weiss, M. (2003) Principals, agents or neither: a qualitative analysis of secondary care commissioning. Paper presented to Health Economists' Study Group Meeting, Leeds.

Bentz, A. (2001) *Information Acquisition and Crowding Out in Regulatory Hierarchies*, CMPO Working Paper, Bristol.

Brennan, G. (1996) Selection and the currency of reward, in R.E. Goodin (ed.) *The Theory of Institutional Design*. Cambridge: Cambridge University Press.

Brennan, G. and Hamlin, A. (2000) *Democratic Devices and Desires*. Cambridge: Cambridge University Press.

Brooks, J., Dor, A. and Wong, H. (1997) Hospital-insurer bargaining: an empirical investigation of appendectomy pricing, *Journal of Health Economics*, 16: 417–34.

Capps, C., Dranove, D., Greenstein, S. and Satterthwaite, M. (2002) Antitrust policy and hospital mergers: recommendations for a new approach, *Antitrust Bulletin*, Winter: 677–714.

Chalkley, M. and Malcomson, J.M. (1998a) Contracting for health services when patient demand does not reflect quality, *Journal of Health Economics*, 17: 1–19.

Chalkley, M. and Malcomson, J.M. (1998b) Contracting for health services with unmonitored quality, *Economic Journal*, 108(449): 1093–110.

Chalkley, M. and Malcomson, J.M. (2000) Government purchasing of health services, in J.P. Newhouse (ed.) *Handbook of Health Economics*. Amsterdam: Elsevier Science.

Chernew, M., Gowrisankaran, G. and Fendrick, M. (2002) Payer type and the returns to bypass surgery: evidence from hospital entry behaviour, *Journal of Health Economics*, 21(3): 451–74.

Cowing, T., Holtman, A. and Powers, S. (1983) Hospital cost analysis: a survey and evaluation of recent studies, *Advances in Health Economics & Health Series Research*, 4: 257–303.

Cowling, K. and Mueller, D. (1978) The social costs of monopoly, *Economic Journal*, 88: 727–48.

Croxson, B., Propper, C. and Perkins, A. (2001) Do doctors respond to financial incentives? UK family doctors and the GP fundholder scheme, *Journal of Public Economics*, 79: 375–98.

Cutler, D. (1995) The incidence of adverse medical outcomes under prospective payment, *Econometrica*, 63(1): 29–50.

Dafny, L. (2003) Entry deterrence in hospital procedure markets: a simple model of learning by doing. IPR/NBER paper.

De Meza, D. and Lockwood, B. (1998) Does asset ownership always motivate managers? Outside options and the property rights theory of the firm, *Quarterly Journal of Economics*, 113: 361–86.

Djankov, S., La Porta, R., Lopez-de Silanes, F. and Shleifer, A. (2001) *The Regulation of Entry*. CEPR discussion paper 2953.

DoH (Department of Health) (2001) *Extending Choice for Patients: A Discussion Document: Proposals for Pilot Schemes to Improve Choice and Provide Faster Treatment*. London: HMSO.

DoH (Department of Health) (2002) *Reforming NHS Financial Flows: Introducing Payment by Results*. London: HMSO.

DoH (Department of Health) (2003) *Standard General Medical Services Contract* (draft). London: DoH.

Dranove, D. and Lindrooth, R. (2003) Hospital consolidation and costs: another look at the evidence, *Journal of Health Economics*, 22(6): 983–97.

Dranove, D. and Ludwick, R. (1999) Competition and pricing by nonprofit hospitals: a reassessment of Lynk's analysis, *Journal of Health Economics*, 18(1): 87–98.

Dranove, D. and White, W. (1994) Recent theory and evidence on competition in hospital markets, *Journal of Economics & Management Strategy*, 3(1): 169–209.

Dusheiko, M., Gravelle, H., Jacobs, R. and Smith, P.C. (2003) *The Effect of Budgets on Doctor Behaviour: Evidence from a Natural Experiment*. University of York Department of Economics and Related Studies Discussion Paper 2003/4; www.york.ac.uk/depts/econ/dp/2003.htm.

Ellis, R.P. and McGuire, T.G. (1990) Optimal payment systems for health services, *Journal of Health Economics*, 9(4): 375–96.

Ellis, R.P. and McGuire, T.G. (1996) Hospital responses to prospective payment: moral hazard, adverse selection and practice-style effects, *Journal of Health Economics*, 15(3): 257–77.

Feldman, R. and Given, R. (1998) HMO mergers and Medicare: the antitrust issues, *Health Economics*, 7(2): 171–4.

Feldman, R., Wisner, C., Dowd, B. and Christianson, J. (1993) An empirical test of competition in the medicare HMO market, in W. White (ed.) *Competitive Approaches to Health Care Reform*. Washington, DC: Urban Institute Press.

Folland, S., Goodman, A.C. and Stano, M. (2001) *The Economics of Health and Health Care*. New Jersey: Prentice-Hall.

Frey, B. (1997) *Not Just for the Money: An Economic Theory of Personal Motivation*. Cheltenham: Edward Elgar.

Fulop, N., Protopsaltis, G., Hutchings, A., King, A., Allen, P., Normand, C. and Walters, R. (2002) Process and impact of mergers of NHS Trusts: multicentre case study and management cost analysis, *British Medical Journal*, 352: 246.

Gandjour, A., Bannenberg, A. and Lauterbach, K.W. (2003) Threshold volumes associated with higher survival in health care: a systematic review, *Medical Care*, 41(10): 1129–41.

Gaynor, M. and Haas-Wilson, D. (1999) Change, consolidation and competition in health care markets, *Journal of Economic Perspectives*, 13(1): 141–64.

Gaynor, M. and Vogt, W. (2000) Antitrust and competition in health care markets, in J.P. Newhouse (ed.) *Handbook of Health Economics*. Amsterdam: Elsevier.

Goddard, M. and Ferguson, B. (1997) *Mergers in the NHS: Made in Heaven or Marriages of Conveniences?* London: Nuffield.

Grossman, S. and Hart, O. (1986) The costs and benefits of ownership: theory of vertical and lateral integration, *Journal of Political Economy*, 94: 691–719.

Guerin, K. (2003) *Encouraging Quality Regulation: Theories and Tools*. New Zealand Treasury Working Paper 03/24.

Haas-Wilson, D. and Gaynor, M. (1998) Physician networks and their implications for competition in health care markets, *Health Economics*, 7(2): 179–82.

Hart, O. (1995) *Firms, Contracts, and Financial Structure*. Oxford: Oxford University Press.

Hart, O. (2003) Incomplete contracts and public ownership: remarks and application to public-private partnerships, *Economic Journal*, 113: C69–C76.

Hart, O. and Moore, J. (1990) Property rights and the nature of the firm, *Journal of Political Economy*, 98: 1119–58.

Hart, O., Shleifer, A. and Vishny, R.W. (1997) The proper scope of government: theory and an application to prisons, *Quarterly Journal of Economics*, 112: 1127–61.

Health Services Journal (2003) 18 September.

Ho, V. and Hamilton, B. (2000) Hospital mergers and acquisitions: does market consolidation harm patients? *Journal of Health Economics*, 19(5): 767–91.

Hodgkin, D. and McGuire, T.M. (1994) Payment levels and hospital response to prospective payment, *Journal of Health Economics*, 13: 1–29.

Holmstrom, B. and Milgrom, P. (1990) Multi-task principle-agent analysis: incentive contracts, asset ownership, and job design, *Journal of Law, Economics and Organization*, 7: 24–52.

James, O. (2000) Regulation inside government: public interest justification and regulatory failures, *Public Administration*, 78(2): 327–43.

Keeler, E., Melnick, G. and Zwanziger, J. (1999) The changing effects of competition on non-profit and for-profit hospital pricing behaviour, *Journal of Health Economics*, 18(1): 69–86.

Klein, B., Crawford, R. and Alchian, A. (1978) Vertical integration, appropriable rents and the competitive contracting process, *Journal of Law and Economics*, 21: 297–326.

Kornai, J., Maskin, E. and Roland, G. (2003) Understanding the soft budget constraint, *Journal of Economic Literature*, XLI (December): 1095–136.

Laffont, J. and Tirole, T. (1991) The politics of government decision-making: a theory of regulatory capture, *Quarterly Journal of Economics*, 106(4): 1089–127.

Le Grand, J. (1997) Knights, knaves, and pawns: human behaviour and social policy, *Journal of Social Policy*, 26(2): 149–69.

Luft, H. (2003) From observing the relationship between volume and outcome to making policy recommendations. Comments of Sheikh. *Medical Care*, 41(10): 1118–22.

Lynk, W. (1995) Nonprofit hospital mergers and the exercise of market power, *Journal of Law and Economics*, 38: 437–61.

Lynk, W. and Neumann, L. (1999) Price and profit, *Journal of Health Economics*, 18(1): 99–105.

Mueller, D.C. (2003) *Public Choice III*. Cambridge: Cambridge University Press.

Newhouse, J., Williams, A., Bennett, B. and Schwartz, W. (1982) Does the geographical distribution of physicians reflect market failure? *Bell Journal of Economics*, 13(2): 493–505.

Newhouse, J.P. (1983) Two prospective difficulties with prospective payment of hospitals, or it's better to be a resident than a patient with a complex problem, *Journal of Health Economics*, 2: 269–74.

Pauly, M.V. (1998) Market power, monopsony and health insurance markets, *Journal of Health Economics*, 7: 111–28.

Peltzman, S. (1989) The economic theory of regulation after a decade of de-regulation, *Brookings Papers on Economic Activity*, 1–41.

Posnett, J. (2001) Are bigger hospitals better? in J. Healy (ed.) *Hospitals in a Changing Europe*. Buckingham: Open University Press.

Propper, C. (1995a) Regulatory reform of the NHS internal market, *Health Economics*, 4: 77–83.

Propper, C. (1995b) Do we need an Ofhealth? *British Medical Journal*, 310: 1618–19.

Propper, C. and Soderlund, N. (1998) Competition in the NHS internal market: an overview of its effects on hospital prices and costs, *Health Economics*, 7: 187–97.

Propper, C., Burgess, S. and Abraham, D. (2002a) *Competition and Quality: Evidence from the Internal Market 1991–1999.* CMPO Working Paper, University of Bristol.

Propper, C., Burgess, S. and Green, K. (2002b) *Does Competition Between Hospitals Improve the Quality of Care? Hospital Death Rates and the Internal Market.* CMPO Working Paper 00/027, University of Bristol.

Rizzo, J. and Sindelar, J. (1996) Optimal regulation of multiply-regulated industries: the case of physician services, *Southern Economics Journal*, 62(April): 966–78.

Sari, N. (2002) Do competition and managed care improve quality? *Health Economics*, 11(7): 571–84.

Secretaries of State for Health (1989) *Working for Patients.* London: HMSO.

Shaw, C. (2001) External assessment of health care, *British Medical Journal*, 322: 851–4.

Sheikh, K. (2003a) Reliability of provider volume and outcome associations for health policy, *Medical Care*, 41(10): 1111–17.

Sheikh, K. (2003b) Sheikh responds to provider volume-patient outcome association and policy by Luft, *Medical Care*, 41(10): 1123–6.

Shleifer, A. (1998) State versus private ownership, *Journal of Economic Perspectives*, 12: 133–50.

Silvia, L. and Leibenlutt, R. (1998) Health economic research and antitrust enforcement, *Health Economics*, 7(2): 163–6.

Sloan (2000) Not-for-profit ownership and hospitals, in J.P. Newhouse (ed.) *Handbook of Health Economics.* Amsterdam: Elsevier.

Smith, P. (2002) Performance management in British health care: will it deliver? *Health Affairs*, 21(3): 103–15.

Sowden, A., Watt, I. and Sheldon, T. (1997) Volume of activity and health care quality: is there a link? in J. Posnett (ed.) *Concentration and Choice in Healthcare.* London: RSM.

Stigler, G. (1971) The theory of economic regulation, *Bell Journal of Economics and Management Science*, 2(1): 1–21.

Tirole, J. (2000) *Incentives and Political Economy.* Cambridge: Cambridge University Press.

Volpp, K., Williams, S., Waldfogel, J., Silber, J., Schwartz, J. and Pauly, M. (2003) Market reform in New Jersey and AMI mortality, *Health Services Research*, 38(2): 515.

Walshe, K. (2002) The rise of regulation in the NHS, *British Medical Journal*, 324: 967–70.

Weisbrod, B.A. (1991) The health care quadrilemma: an essay on techno-logical change, insurance, quality of care, and cost containment, *Journal of Economic Literature*, 29(2): 523–52.

6

EFFICIENCY MEASUREMENT IN HEALTH CARE: RECENT DEVELOPMENTS, CURRENT PRACTICE AND FUTURE RESEARCH

Rowena Jacobs and Andrew Street

INTRODUCTION

In 1994 the *Journal of Health Economics* (*JHE*) published a set of papers and commentaries delivered at a symposium on efficiency and frontier analysis in health care. Commenting on the material, the *JHE*'s editor concluded: 'I am doubtful that the regulator can recover "true" or efficient cost or production parameters from observed data with any degree of precision' (Newhouse 1994). Since then, not a single article relating to this line of research has appeared in the *JHE*, presumably, in part at least, because of the criticisms made by the symposium's three commentators (Dor 1994; Newhouse 1994; Skinner 1994). Whether explicit or implicit, this editorial decision might be defended on two grounds. First, the *JHE* may be an inappropriate outlet for research of this nature, irrespective of advances made in efficiency measurement since 1994. We support this position. Second, if no degree of precision is possible, efficiency studies in health care are unworthy of publication altogether and should not be used to inform policy. We reject this more damning indictment.

Irrespective of their supposed influence on *JHE* editorial policy, the criticisms raised at the symposium have done little to stem wider policy interest in efficiency measurement. The authors and commentators at the symposium envisaged that frontier analysis would be used primarily to inform reimbursement policy, with regulators perhaps implementing budget reductions by the amount of measured inefficiency (Newhouse 1994). There are examples of such applications in other sectors. For instance, the UK water regulator has employed frontier techniques to inform price setting (Office of Water Trading 1999).

More commonly, though, frontier analysis has been embraced by policymakers keen to enhance the accountability of organizations that have public sector responsibilities. This drive for improved accountability arrangements stems from a general desire to ensure value for money in the use of public funds, and the Chief Secretary of the UK Treasury has stated that efficiency analysis has wide potential application across all public services (Public Services Productivity Panel 2004).

Regulators assessing the relative performance of organizations with multiple and complex objectives may draw on a suite of individual performance indicators to assist them. Separate performance indicators have many benefits. They focus on specific aspects of performance, are readily measured and validated, and are easy to interpret (in isolation, at least). However, there are two major drawbacks to using individual performance indicators. First, they provide only an indirect or partial indication of overall performance. Second, they may provide conflicting messages: an organization that appears to do well on one indicator may perform less successfully when considering another. It is not straightforward to draw conclusions about overall organizational performance from a range of performance indicators. The techniques of efficiency measurement promise to address these shortcomings by constructing an objective function, which specifies the relationship between multiple objectives (or the performance indicators used to measure them), and then produces a single summary measure of efficiency based on the shortfall between observed and predicted performance.

In this review of efficiency measurement in health care we evaluate how these single indices are constructed. We start with the three papers and accompanying commentaries presented at the *JHE* symposium. We provide a description of the two techniques employed in the papers, namely Stochastic Frontier Analysis (SFA) and Data Envelopment Analysis (DEA). In describing the techniques, we summarize criticisms raised in the commentaries, and provide an overview of subsequent advances made in this area, and an indication as to whether or not the criticisms raised at the symposium still hold. We suggest that, irrespective of methodological advances, inferences about efficiency from such studies should still be drawn with caution. We conclude by defending the *JHE*'s (implicit) editorial policy, and suggest an alternative way forward for organizational performance assessment that strikes a balance between the construction of a single summary measure and the use of multiple performance indicators.

THE *JHE* SYMPOSIUM: THE PAPERS AND TECHNIQUES

Three papers were published from the symposium, two of which employed SFA (Vitaliano and Toren 1994a; Zuckerman *et al.* 1994), while the other utilized DEA (Kooreman 1994a). All three were cross-sectional analyses, although one separately analysed two years' worth of data (Vitaliano and Toren 1994a). Many of the criticisms made in the commentaries (summarized in Table 6.1) are inherent to cross-sectional data and might be alleviated if longitudinal (panel) data were available. As such, we describe both cross-sectional and longitudinal applications of the methods.

Table 6.1 Criticisms raised at *JHE* symposium, and subsequently

Criticism	Author	Response
DEA & SFA: difficulty of measuring output, particularly quality	Newhouse (1994)	Still holds, but endemic to all health services research
DEA & SFA: misinterpretation as a result of model misspecification and omitted variables	Newhouse (1994) and Dor (1994)	Still holds
DEA & SFA: casemix controls (e.g. DRGs) inadequate	Newhouse (1994)	Some advances in most health care systems
DEA & SFA: large number of parameters, particularly in functional forms that include higher powers	Newhouse (1994)	Ways of collapsing data to manageable numbers of parameters without losing information
SFA: difficulty in handling multiple outputs	Kooreman (1994a)	Estimate SFA cost function; use DEA
DEA: failure to account for statistical error	Newhouse (1994) and Dor (1994)	Still holds

SFA x-section: non-testable assumptions about distribution of inefficiency	Newhouse (1994)	Conduct sensitivity analysis; estimate FE panel data model
SFA x-section: assumption of normality of statistical error	Skinner (1994)	Use panel data
SFA x-section: assumption that skewness indicates inefficiency	Skinner (1994)	Use panel data
SFA x-section: cannot compute inefficiency independently of statistical error	Dor (1994)	Use panel data
SFA x-section: no test of endogeneity of outputs in cost function	Dor (1994)	Use panel data
DEA: second stage analysis – no strong theoretical justification for stage at which variables included	Dor (1994)	Second stage analysis to be avoided altogether because efficiency scores are serially correlated
SFA FE panel: requires observation of all time invariant factors	Dor (1994)	Estimate RE model
SFA RE panel: requires assumption about distribution of efficiency	–	Still holds
SFA panel: efficiency estimates contaminated by unobserved heterogeneity	Dor (1994)	Estimate 'true' FE and RE models (Greene forthcoming)
SFA panel: efficiency assumed time-invariant	Dor (1994)	More flexible specifications allow time-varying efficiency (Linna 1998)
DEA & SFA: inadequate theory of cost-minimizing behaviour	Dor (1994)	Still holds
DEA & SFA: flexible output weights invalidate comparisons across organizations	–	Weights should be generated as part of separate analytical process, informed by purpose of analysis

Stochastic Frontier Analysis (SFA)

The papers by Zuckerman *et al.* (1994) and Vitaliano and Toren (1994a) applied SFA to cost functions. Zuckerman *et al.* used 1600 US hospitals and Vitaliano and Toren used 607 nursing homes in New York state. It is more common to estimate a cost, rather than production, function because of the difficulties in constructing a single measure of production for organizations that produce multiple outputs. We shall return to this problem in due course. When estimating a cost function using cross-sectional data, the stochastic frontier can be written as (Coelli *et al.* 1998):

$$y_i = a + x_i \beta + \varepsilon_i = a + x_i \beta + (v_i + u_i) \quad i = 1, \ldots, N \tag{1}$$

where y_i is the (total or unit) cost of production of the ith hospital in either linear or logarithmic form; a is a constant; x_i is a vector of explanatory variables for the ith organization that are unrelated to efficiency but thought to explain differences in cost; and β is a vector of unknown parameters. The crucial difference between this formulation and a standard neoclassical cost (or production) function is the treatment of the error term, ε_i, which is usually expected to satisfy the classical conventions for regression analysis, but is here decomposed into two components. The rationale for this departure is that, in contexts where inefficiency is likely to be present, the classical error term ε_i will be capturing both standard statistical noise, v_i, and within sample inefficiency, u_i.

The dual specification of the residual in SFA is defended on the grounds that each component reflects an economically distinct disturbance (Aigner *et al.* 1977). v_i can be interpreted as representing stochastic (random) events not under control of the organizations, such as climatic conditions, random equipment failure, errors in identifying or measuring explanatory variables, or omitted variables (Timmer 1971; Aigner *et al.* 1977; Greene 1993). In the hospital sector, for instance, these stochastic disturbances might be unanticipated expenditures for hospital repairs, unexpected winter pressure on beds arising from cold weather, a temporary local outbreak of disease, a suddenly interrupted source of supply or unexpected personnel problems (Folland and Hofler 2001).

u_i is a non-negative error term accounting for the cost of inefficiency in production, capturing how far the ith hospital operates above the cost frontier, and incorporates both technical and allocative inefficiency. The estimation problem is how to locate the frontier and how to separate inefficiency from statistical noise. In cross-sectional

analysis this is achieved by imposing assumptions on how inefficiency and statistical noise are distributed, so that it is possible to
extract estimates of u_i conditional upon v_i. Following classical conventions v_i is assumed to be independent and identically distributed
with zero mean and variance σ^2_v. Within-sample inefficiency, u_i is
assumed to be skewed, with values bounded to lie at, or above, zero
(no inefficiency). Standard software packages provide various distributional options, including the half-normal, truncated-normal,
exponential and gamma distributions. There is no economic rationale for favouring one distribution over another, although it may be
possible to choose on statistical grounds (Schmidt 1985). While there
has been some debate in the literature over the choice of distribution
(Vitaliano and Toren 1994b), in practice this choice of distribution is
of secondary importance, as results are generally far more sensitive
to other decisions made in the estimation process.

More critical to the technique – and the main focus of Skinner's
(1994) symposium commentary – is that, for estimation to proceed,
the composite error term, ε_i must be skewed, with skewness being
taken as evidence of inefficiency within the sample (Schmidt and Lin
1984). In situations where ε_i are normally distributed, all residual
variance is interpreted as being attributable to statistical noise and,
hence, it is not possible to detect inefficiency (Wagstaff 1989). The
requirement that the composite residual is skewed makes it difficult
to assess the appropriateness of the underlying model, because
standard econometric procedures that rely on tests of the classical
error term cannot be applied in the cross-sectional SFA context. In
this context, it simply has to be *assumed* that the model is correctly
specified and that skewness arises solely from inefficiency, rather
than an inappropriate functional form, omitted variables or
heteroscedasticity.

The problem of applying standard model specification tests is further compounded in the SFA context because of the purpose of the
analysis. In most situations in which econometric analysis is applied,
the research interest is in estimating *average* effects from the sample
data. In contrast, in SFA the purpose is often to extract *individual*
estimates of inefficiency for each organization. This difference in
emphasis means that we cannot apply the usual statistical criteria to
decide whether or not to include a variable. While its effect may not
be statistically significant across the sample as a whole, it may be
highly material in explaining observed costs (or output) for a select
number of organizations. By excluding this variable on the basis of
statistical insignificance, it is likely that much of its effect will be

captured by u_i and, for those few organizations to which it matters, their inefficiency will be overestimated.

Unable to rely on statistical tests, model specification must be guided by economic theory and the appropriate theoretical framework is likely to be dependent on the purpose of the analysis. In the health care sector, the appropriate specification of hospital cost, or production, functions has long been a source of controversy, and it is not surprising that the SFA literature mirrors this larger debate (Breyer 1987). The two SFA papers presented at the symposium both estimate models drawn from the neoclassical theory of the firm, with costs being a function of output levels and factor prices, although both specifications include additional variables that have been described as ad hoc by other commentators on the wider literature (Breyer 1987). The problem with using a specification based on the theory of the firm for efficiency analysis is that most of the variables are likely to be endogenous, resulting in parameter estimates being biased and inconsistent. Both sets of symposium authors acknowledged this problem and tried either to correct for it (e.g. by instrumentation) or to explain it away. Moreover, the endogeneity does not relate solely to the question of whether high costs are caused by higher outputs (or vice versa), but also to the question of what aspects of the production technology the organization has control over.

Given the shortcomings of cross-sectional data, both Skinner and Dor, in their commentaries, recommended the analysis of longitudinal data, in which organizations are observed over several time periods. Repeated observations of the same organization make it possible to control for unobservable organization-specific attributes and, thereby, to extract more reliable parameter estimates, both of the explanatory variables and the efficiency term. The panel data model takes the following general form (Kumbhakar and Lovell 2000),

$$y_{it} = a + \beta x_{it} + u_{it} + v_{it}, \quad u_{it} \geq 0 \tag{2}$$

where t indexes time, and u_{it} captures inefficiency. If inefficiency can be assumed constant over time, it is possible to perform estimation using two estimators commonly applied to panel data: the fixed effects and the random effects approaches.

The fixed effects estimator is equivalent to adding a dummy variable for each organization, and this generates a set of organization-specific constants, $a_i = a + u_i$ (Schmidt and Sickles 1984). The estimated frontier, $\hat{a}$, is located by assuming that the organization with the lowest constant value is fully efficient (in the case of the cost function), such that $\hat{a} = \min_i(a_i)$. Individual time-invariant estimates of inefficiency, $\hat{u}_i$, can be derived from $\hat{u}_i = a_i - \min_i(\hat{a}_i)$.

The fixed effects estimator relies on there being sufficient within-hospital variation over time. In other words, the value of x must vary for individual organizations from one period to the next. In particular, if there are organizational factors that explain costs, but which do not vary over time – such as the operating environment – their influence will be captured by the organizational-specific term, a_i. Thus, the fixed effect estimator fails to distinguish between time invariant heterogeneity and inefficiency.

To avoid this, Pitt and Lee (1981) advocated using the random effects estimator, which necessitates imposing a distributional assumption on u, and, as in the cross-sectional context, both half-normal (Pitt and Lee 1981) and truncated normal (Battese and Coelli 1988) distributions have been proposed. Essentially, the random effects model assumes that organizational effects are random draws from a population. Accordingly, the estimator has the advantage of utilizing information about variation within individual organizations over time (within-variation) and across different organizations in the sample (between-variation). This makes the random effects more efficient than the fixed effects estimator. However, given that it is usual to estimate these types of model to generate inferences about individual organizations, the assumption that the effects are random draws from a population may be unwarranted, implying that the fixed effects estimator is to be preferred (Rice and Jones 1997). Additionally, the fixed effects estimator will be favoured in those circumstances where the explanatory variables are correlated with the organization-specific effects. The Hausman test is used to discriminate between the two estimators (Hausman 1978).

Recent research has focused on enriching these standard panel data models for use in efficiency analysis. One avenue has been to estimate stochastic frontier models with a time varying inefficiency component, for instance by allowing the intercept of the model to change so that individual effects can evolve over time (Cornwell *et al.* 1990; Linna 1998). These models of time-varying technical efficiency require the imposition of strong assumptions about the temporal pattern in which technical efficiency may vary across organizations (Kumbhakar 1990). Another approach has been to better separate unobserved organizational heterogeneity from inefficiency (Farsi *et al.* 2003; Greene forthcoming). Again, this requires distributional assumptions to be made about the form of heterogeneity.

Irrespective of whether or not panel data are available, the ability of SFA to identify organizational efficiency precisely depends crucially on whether inefficiency and statistical noise, u and v, are independent and/or whether there is spillover across the partitioned error term. The problem is that a non-negative term may be observed for a variety of reasons other than inefficiency. Stigler suggested that supposedly 'inefficient' behaviour might be observed because of an incorrectly specified objective function, a failure to account for all relevant inputs and a lack of recognition of the constraints on the production process (Stigler 1976). These factors may explain one-sided disturbances in the stochastic frontier framework (Dopuch and Gupta 1997). Unobserved characteristics of acute hospitals, for instance, that may contribute to a significant non-negative term include the following:

- 'Correct' specification of the objective function depends, of course, on whose objectives are afforded primacy. Society, regulators and hospital management teams may not share the same goals, in which case they will have different definitions of what constitutes efficient behaviour. Strategies to reduce costs by engaging in risk selection or skimping on care are examples where managerial objectives may be socially sub-optimal (Ellis 1998).
- The pursuit of multiple objectives in the health sector further complicates interpretation. Actions that give rise to 'cost inefficiency' may be efficient means of meeting an alternative objective. For example, one possible objective might be for hospitals to provide care in a timely fashion. In order to be able to admit emergency patients immediately, hospitals must keep some capacity in reserve, simply because the daily arrival process governing the presentation of such patients is unpredictable (Joskow 1980; Bagust *et al.* 1999). If it is considered important that hospitals do not turn emergency patients away because beds are unavailable, there is an argument for incorporating this explicitly in the hospital's objective function. Moreover, there are likely to be systematic differences across hospitals in their ability to meet the objective. In order to offer a similar probability of admission, smaller hospitals will have to maintain a greater amount of reserve capacity than larger hospitals (Joskow 1980). The inevitable cost disadvantage that this imposes might be labelled incorrectly as inefficiency.
- Hospitals face diverse constraints on their operating process. For example, those operating in environments where community and

primary care is underdeveloped will be more constrained in their ability to discharge patients to more appropriate settings and will face higher costs as a result (Fernández and Forder 2002).

• Coding practices may be less accurate in particular types of hospital. Hospitals with a more varied and complex case mix may find that the complexity of their activity is under-reported because coding systems are insufficiently sophisticated, or because medical records personnel code imprecisely the less common diagnoses or procedures.

• Accounting practices may vary, if hospitals with a more diverse set of activities – such as those engaged in teaching and research – are able to exercise discretion about what costs to attribute to patient care services.

As these examples suggest, the problems of interpretation are intrinsically bound up with model specification and accurate observation of all relevant data (Dopuch and Gupta 1997). Given the comments made earlier about the difficulty of applying standard statistical tests to assess model specification, theoretical considerations are of paramount importance. Specifications of SFA models tend to fall into one of two groups: those that are based on the neoclassical theory of the firm and those that are drawn from regulatory theory.

The former type of specification models the production process in relation to input use, with the production function summarizing a technical relationship between maximum output attainable for different combinations of all possible factors of production. However, this neoclassical application may be questionable, particularly if inefficiency is thought to derive from sub-optimal decisions about the level and mix of inputs – which may be considered key elements over which organizations enjoy discretion. By specifying inputs among the explanatory variables, incorrect utilization decisions are captured in the associated parameter estimates.

Specifications that appeal to the theory of regulation are motivated by the recognition that regulators of industries that face little competition often wish to exert downward pressure on costs by regulating prices, setting efficiency targets or simply 'naming and shaming' the organizations into making a response. The regulator may wish to examine output or costs in order to be able to make inferences about the levels of effort applied by the organizations being regulated. Below average costs may be observed in organizations that expend more effort in searching for, and applying, efficient modes of operation. However, observed costs may not be related to efficiency alone, particularly if firms face different operating environments, or other influences on their costs that are not subject to managerial control. To be able to draw accurate inferences about the relationship between output or costs and effort, the regulator would want to include variables in the model that control for these exogenous influences (Schleifer 1985). In fact, it has been argued that if the objective of the exercise is to make inferences about relative efficiency, a necessary condition is that all variables included as regressors are exogenous to managerial influence (Giuffrida *et al.* 2000). The choice for the analyst, then, is to determine what are valid exogenous variables and over what timeframe the constraints are binding. Obviously, such constraints will be highly context-specific and, in all likelihood, an area of contention between the regulator and the regulated organizations.

What constitutes the appropriate theoretical framework would appear to be a fruitful avenue for future research and, indeed, in his commentary, Dor (1994) suggested directions that might be taken for the analysis of non-minimum cost behaviour. As yet, though, this fundamental issue has received limited attention in the literature on efficiency analysis, and further research is required.

Data envelopment analysis (DEA)

The third paper published from the symposium applied DEA to assess the efficiency of all 320 nursing homes in the Netherlands using data from 1989. Unlike SFA, a significant drawback of DEA is that, as Dor remarked: 'unfortunately . . . all random noise in the DEA is lumped together with the true inefficiency, making the resulting inefficiency scores suspect' (Dor 1994: 329). In some circumstances, it may be possible to sustain an argument that there is no measurement error. Indeed, Kooreman defended the application in the nursing home setting, stating that 'since the survey forms have been filled out by the administrative staff of the nursing homes, who may be assumed to be well-informed about their home, measurement errors are likely to be small' (Kooreman 1994a: 305). This assumption may have less foundation in larger, or more complex, organizational contexts (such as hospitals), and may be further undermined if those responsible for data collection change their reporting behaviour in the knowledge that the information they provide is to be used for the purpose of efficiency assessment or reimbursement.

The failure to account for statistical noise remains a fundamental shortcoming of the DEA technique and may explain why Kooreman's paper received limited attention in the symposium's accompanying commentaries. Nevertheless, DEA has become the most widely used technique to measure efficiency in the health care sector (Hollingsworth *et al.* 1999).

One major facet of the appeal of the DEA method, based on the work of Farrell (1957) and developed subsequently by Charnes *et al.* (1978), is that it is intuitively simple: it is based on the straightforward notion that, in producing a given level of output, organizations that employ less input are more efficient. Another attractive feature is that, unlike SFA, there is no computational difficulty in applying the technique to a multiple output context.

Organizational efficiency is defined as the ratio of the weighted sum of each organization's outputs divided by a weighted sum of its inputs (Smith 1998). DEA can be applied to the analysis of organizations observed over multiple periods by constructing the Malmquist index (Coelli *et al.* 1998). For simplicity, though, we shall describe the technique as applied to cross-sectional data. The comments apply irrespective of the longitudinal nature of the data. In the single input-output context, technical efficiency for organization i is defined as $EFF_i = Q_i/L_i$. In the case of multiple inputs and outputs, the measure of technical efficiency is expressed as the ratio of a weighted sum of outputs to a weighted sum of inputs,

$$EFF_i = \frac{\sum_{f=1}^{F} m_f Q_{fi}}{\sum_{g=1}^{G} n_g L_{gi}} \tag{3}$$

where f is an index of outputs, $f = 1 \ldots F$, and g is an index of inputs, $g = 1 \ldots G$ and m_f and n_g are the weights attached to output f and input g respectively. DEA assigns weights to each output and each input, derived by examining all linear combinations of comparable (peer) organizations that produce at least as much as the organization under consideration.

Assuming constant returns to scale, the maximization problem for organization D, in a sample of i organizations, can be expressed as (Hollingsworth *et al.* 1999):

$$\max EFF_D = \frac{\displaystyle\sum_{f=1}^{F} m_f\, Q_{fD}}{\displaystyle\sum_{g=1}^{G} n_g\, L_{gD}}$$

subject to $\hspace{8cm}$ (4)

$$\frac{\displaystyle\sum_{f=1}^{F} m_f\, Q_{fi}}{\displaystyle\sum_{g=1}^{G} n_g\, L_{gi}} \leq 1, \qquad m_f,\ n_g > 0$$

The constraints state that the ratio of weighted output over weighted input must lie between 0 and 1 for all organizations in the sample.

For computational ease, and because relative, rather than absolute, values are of interest, it is usual to constrain either inputs or outputs to equal unity. Efficiency can be defined as either output-oriented (maximizing outputs per unit of input) or input-oriented (minimizing inputs per unit of output). The choice of orientation depends on the analyst's view over which parameters it is believed organizations exercise control. For instance, hospital specialties may face a fixed quantity of inputs in any given period. Subject to this resource constraint, managers must decide how many patients to treat. This would imply that technical efficiency is measured by considering the extent to which outputs can be expanded proportionately without altering the quantity of inputs. This suggests an output-oriented measure of efficiency. In contrast, if, say, contractual arrangements are specified in terms of a target number of patients treated, the managerial problem might be better formulated by considering how much input quantities could be reduced while still achieving the output target. This would imply an input orientation to the problem. Hence, if the problem is reformulated so that the organization aims to maximize a weighted sum of outputs, the previous equation is rewritten as:

$$\max EFF_D = \sum_{f=1}^{F} m_f\, Q_{fD}$$

subject to $\hspace{8cm}$ (5)

$$\sum_{g=1}^{G} n_g L_{gD} = 1, \quad \sum_{f=1}^{F} m_f Q_{fD} - \sum_{g=1}^{G} n_g L_{gi} \le 0, \quad m_f, n_g > 0$$

The choice of orientation does not affect which observations are identified as fully efficient since the models will estimate exactly the same frontier (Coelli *et al.* 1998). However, output- and input-oriented models will generate different measures of technical efficiency for organizations that do not lie on the frontier, unless it can be assumed that there are constant returns to scale. The DEA method considers whether efficiency estimates are conditional upon the scale of operation (Banker *et al.* 1984). This entails allowing the production frontier to exhibit variable returns to scale. The assumption of constant returns to scale can be relaxed by adding a parameter S to the maximization problem:

$$\max EFF_D = \sum_{f=1}^{F} m_f Q_{fD} + S$$

subject to (6)

$$\sum_{g=1}^{G} n_g L_{gD} = 1, \quad \sum_{f=1}^{F} m_f Q_{fD} - \sum_{g=1}^{G} n_g L_{gi} + S \le 0, \quad m_f, n_g > 0$$

When $S = 0$ the frontier is constrained to exhibit constant returns, $S < 0$ allows decreasing returns, and if S is unrestricted then variable returns are allowed. The efficiency frontier takes a 'piecewise-linear' form, in that it comprises straight-line segments that join up the outermost observations. Invariably, the assumption of variable returns to scale will result in higher estimates of efficiency than constant returns to scale, because the frontier envelopes the data more tightly. The approach known as Free Disposal Hull (FDH) analysis allows an even closer fit of the frontier to the data, by fitting a piecewise linear function that is permitted to display non-increasing segments (in the case of the production frontier) (Tulkens 1993). FDH generates a frontier that increases in a step-like fashion. However, it is difficult to think of any economic rationale for why a frontier would display such characteristics.

Organizations with the largest ratio of outputs to inputs are deemed to lie on and, therefore, define the efficiency frontier. This frontier will envelope all other organizations, making it possible to calculate their efficiency relative to this surface (Charnes *et al.* 1994).

The frontier, then, is defined solely in relation to the extreme observations. This avoids having to appeal to theoretical considerations, other than the notion of scale economies, in defining the shape and location of the frontier. But this pure empiricism makes the technique highly sensitive to the influence of outliers, thereby compounding the failure to recognize the possibility of measurement error. For instance, in standard applications of DEA, if an organization is unique in producing a single type of output it will be defined as lying on the efficiency frontier, even if, in fact, it uses excessive inputs to produce its other outputs.

One of the reasons why the technique is sensitive to unusual observations stems from the derivation of the output and input weights. In most applications of DEA, rather than being input and output specific, the weights are allowed to vary across organizations. The justification for unrestricted weights is that it allows each organization to be seen in the best possible light. For each organization, DEA computes all possible sets of these weights and chooses those weights that assign the highest efficiency score (Pedraja-Chaparro *et al.* 1997). This means, at the extreme, that it is possible for an organization to be considered fully efficient simply by assigning a zero weight to an output on which it performs poorly. The problem with this flexibility is that it undermines the statements that can be drawn about relative efficiency. Do differential efficiency scores result from different choices about the output-input mix, or from different valuations of outputs and inputs? The consequence is that, in contexts where organizational flexibility about these relative valuations is permissible, it is inappropriate to use the DEA scores to make statements about relative efficiency. If estimates of relative performance are required, it is necessary to impose a standard objective function across all organizations, and this implies a standard set of output and input weights.

There has been some attention to rules for restricting the flexibility of weight variations (Allen *et al.* 1997) and various authors have suggested ways of imposing restrictions on the weights, including Roll *et al.* (1991), Dyson and Thanassoulis (1988), Thompson *et al.* (1990), and Wong and Beasley (1990). However, efforts have been confined mainly to technical considerations, rather than being informed by the purposes of the analysis (Pedraja-Chaparro *et al.* 1997). If DEA is being employed to inform policy, the weights should reflect political judgements about the relative importance of different outputs, and about the relative opportunity cost of the inputs used. Selection of these weights cannot then be subsumed within DEA, but needs to be undertaken as a separate exercise.

An ongoing debate among proponents of DEA is the matter of how to control for the fact that organizations operate in diverse environmental contexts, and that in many applications this ought to be taken into account when undertaking analysis. Broadly, two possibilities are available, neither of which is satisfactory. First, variables reflecting the operating environment are included in the DEA problem, as an additional set of constraints. The problem here is that many organizations face unique environments and are automatically deemed fully efficient. Thus DEA loses much discriminatory power. The second possibility is to analyse the efficiency scores in a second-stage econometric analysis. This is what Kooreman (1994a) did, and there are countless other applications of DEA that do the same, usually by specifying a regression model that recognizes the truncated nature of the dependent variable (i.e. the efficiency scores). There is a seeming inconsistency in first rejecting econometric techniques in favour of non-parametric techniques and then re-embracing them in a second-stage analysis. Dor (1994) also argues that there is little theoretical justification for the choice of variables at each stage. More critically, though, it is rarely recognized that the parameter estimates and the standard errors from these second-stage regressions are inherently biased. This bias originates from the fact that the efficiency scores derived from the DEA programme are serially correlated, thereby violating the classical assumption that observations are independent. This undermines standard approaches to inference, and implies that caution should be exercised when interpreting these second-stage results (Simar and Wilson 2002).

CAUTIOUS APPLICATION IS ADVISABLE

From the above discussion it might be thought that, indeed, the problems of efficiency measurement are so significant as to invalidate this entire field of research. But it is not surprising that efficiency is difficult to measure, being, like wisdom, beauty and love, a quality about which there are inevitable definitional and quantitative challenges. Economics would indeed be a dismal science were it dismissive of such qualities, simply because they are not precisely quantifiable.

Actually, not only is efficiency difficult to observe and quantify, but there is dispute over what constitutes appropriate specifications of health service outputs – or, more generally, health service object-ives. Indeed, the overriding rationale for Newhouse's (1994) rejection of frontier analysis appears to stem from the difficulties in specifying health care outputs, along both quantitative and qualitative dimen-sions. Measurement of quality has indeed often been conspicuously absent in efficiency studies – though recently various authors have explicitly incorporated measures of quality into the objective func-tion (Puig-Junoy 1998; Maniadakis *et al.* 1999). But it can hardly be claimed that specifying health care outputs is a vexing question solely for those involved in efficiency analysis, as it is pervasive across the spectrum of health care research, from the measurement of patient outcomes in clinical trials to the identification of health sys-tem outputs for the purpose of constructing national accounts. This difficulty is particularly acute for efficiency measurement where, as Newhouse remarked, SFA and DEA are better suited to analysis of industries with 'readily measurable, homogenous output' (1994: 321).

Unlike DEA, SFA is ill-suited to the consideration of multiple outputs, but two methods of handling the problem have been developed. The first, and most obvious, is to estimate a cost (rather than production) function, using duality theory to argue that the two are equivalent. However, duality holds only if cost-minimizing behaviour can be assumed, which is probably not the case given that the purpose of the exercise is to identify departures from cost mini-mization. The second approach is to condition one of the outputs on the others in some way (Coelli and Perelman 1996; Morrison *et al.* 2000). But, as with DEA, this imposes an implicit set of weights on the outputs. In the SFA context, the output weights correspond to sample average values and, again, this may not be appropriate when sub-optimal behaviour is thought prevalent. Whenever a single index of performance is to be generated for the sake of making compara-tive statements, the issue of weighting the various objectives arises. Multi-dimensional SFA and DEA cannot avoid this fundamental problem, although the issue is often obscured in the application.

Another problem in using the techniques is that there is rarely agreement between the results of SFA and DEA, even for fairly simple production techniques and when the underlying models are equivalent (Thanassoulis 1993; Linna 1998; Giuffrida and Gravelle 2001; Jacobs 2001). Any discrepancies are due to differences in how the methods establish the location and shape of the frontier, and in determining how far individual observations lie above it. In SFA, statistical criteria might be used to differentiate between the appropriateness of alternative theoretical functional relationships to describe costs in particular datasets. In the absence of statistical discrimination, if the rankings of organizational efficiency estimates are sensitive to the functional form applied, it would be inadvisable to draw firm conclusions about their relative efficiency.

Advocates of DEA would argue that the problems of providing a prior specification of functional form can be avoided by applying the non-parametric technique. Here the frontier is defined solely by the data: the outermost observations, given the scale of operation, are defined as efficient. As such, the frontier is positioned and shaped by the data, not by theoretical considerations. Consequently, DEA is highly flexible (completely so, in the case of the FDH variant), with the frontier moulding itself to the data. Thus, if the results of DEA and (say) a logarithmic stochastic frontier model correspond, it could be concluded that the frontier truly displays logarithmic properties for the data analysed. Where the results deviate, this may be because the monotonic assumptions of the SFA model are too restrictive, and DEA is able to account for segments of the frontier where a smooth relationship is not apparent in the data. For those who approach efficiency measurement from an empirical rather than theoretical standpoint, the flexibility of functional form offered by DEA would seem an attractive feature of the technique.

While DEA might be thought to win out over the SFA method in terms of flexibility, this is offset by its use of a selective amount of data to estimate individual efficiency scores. DEA generates efficiency scores for each organization by comparing it only to peers that produce a comparable mix of outputs. This has two implications. First, if any output is unique to an organization, it will have no peers with which to make a comparison, irrespective of the fact that it may produce other outputs in common. An absence of peers results in the automatic assignation of full efficiency for the organization under consideration. Second, when assigning an inefficiency score to an observation not lying on the frontier, only its peers are considered, with information pertaining to the remainder of the sample discarded. In contrast, SFA appeals to the full sample information when estimating relative efficiency. In addition to making greater use of the available data, this facet of the estimation procedure will make individual efficiency estimates more robust in the presence of outlier observations and to the presence of atypical input/output combinations.

Given that there can be no clear grounds for preferring either SFA or DEA estimation, the question arises as to how to use the techniques. Kooreman (1994b) suggests that DEA and SFA are complementary tools that can be used in conjunction with each other as devices to signal the presence of inefficiency, and to take action as appropriate, perhaps by sacking the management. We agree that the methods may be useful as signalling devices of inefficiency, but contend that the signals are too noisy to justify severe sanctions, and that it is probably best not to expect the models to yield definitive statements about relative efficiency. Rather, they should be considered tools of exploratory data analysis. For any given dataset, comparison of the DEA and SFA efficiency estimates will allow organizations to be sorted into three groups. First, there will be a group where relative efficiency is sensitive to the choice of technique. It would be inadvisable to draw firm conclusions about their actual level of relative efficiency. Second, there will be organizations that appear efficient whichever technique is adopted, and however the models are specified. Further analysis of the working practices of these organizations may be informative if a purpose or byproduct of the exercise is to share best practice. However, because DEA assigns full efficiency to unusual observations (i.e. those which do not have peers), the method may be labelling organizations as efficient when it would be more appropriate to consider them as outliers. It may not be good practice to make policy recommendations on the basis of outlier behaviour. Finally, there will be a group of organizations that always appear inefficient, irrespective of the measurement technique employed. These might be deserving of greater scrutiny to ascertain the reasons why their performance appears to fall short of that of their counterparts.

A more drastic implication of the lack of consistency in the results derived from DEA and SFA would be to dispense with a single efficiency measure as a summary of overall performance and, instead, assess efficiency on individual objectives. The use of a single summary measure is appealing to external bodies because it promises to simplify the assessment process. Superficially it appears much less demanding to make judgements on the basis of a single measure than to have to grapple with several dimensions of performance. But, in addition to the problem of how to weight different objectives, the use of a single measure implies that important information may be 'lost'. From an organizational perspective, if performance assessment is to engender behavioural change, it is essential that the assessment technique provides clear messages (Nutley and Smith 1998). The use of a single measure carries the risk that important information will be difficult to access. It is not immediately apparent to organizations how they perform on the specific performance dimensions that have been amalgamated into the single index and, hence, where they should focus their attention. Moreover, if the index is based on unconstrained weights, organizations will not be able to separately identify sub-optimality in performance from differences in the relative values placed upon objectives.

However, rejection of a single efficiency index does not imply a retreat back to the use of a suite of separate performance indicators. A major drawback of using separate indicators is that this approach fails to recognize that organizational achievement may be correlated across objectives. This correlation may be positive, if progress against one indicator simultaneously advances another, perhaps because good management promotes all-round performance. But the correlation may be negative if trade-offs are involved, such as when resources have to be diverted from one activity in order to meet some other objective. Rather, a middle way between the analysis of objectives in isolation and the creation of a single index may be appropriate. This involves estimating multivariate models, using seemingly unrelated regression (SUR) techniques, which treat each objective as part of a system of equations but allow for correlations across objectives (Hauck and Street 2004; Bailey and Hewson forthcoming). A major advantage of the SUR method for performance assessment in the context of multiple objectives is that it does not require us to weight objectives because information on relative performance is provided specifically for each objective.

An extension of this approach would be the estimation of multivariate multi-level models, which involves simultaneously modelling several objectives, but in addition recognizing the existence of clustering in the data. Focusing on the hierarchical nature of the data enables researchers to understand at what levels variations in performance are occurring (Browne and Rasbash 2001).

CONCLUSIONS

We started this review by offering two possible defences for why the *JHE* has published no papers on efficiency measurement since the 1994 symposium. The *JHE* is perhaps not the most appropriate outlet for research of this nature. Most of the advances in efficiency measurement made since the symposium, of which there have been many, are general to this field of research, rather than specific to the health care sector. Hence, journals with a more general readership, such as the *Journal of Econometrics* or the *Journal of Productivity Analysis*, are more appropriate for reporting (say) improvements to statistical methodology.

The more damning critique is that, if no degree of precision is possible, efficiency studies are unworthy of publication altogether and should not be used to inform policy. This can be countered on two fronts. First, as Hadley and Zuckerman (1994) argued in their response to the symposium commentaries, the primary purpose of efficiency measurement should not be to extract precise point estimates. Rather, such studies should be used as a form of exploratory data analysis, allowing screening of observations to identify those where further scrutiny of their working practices may be warranted. To support this application of the techniques, analysts should test the sensitivity of their results and provide confidence statements around their point estimates (Horrace and Schmidt 1996; Jensen 2000; Street 2003).

Second, clearly there are areas where further research in the field is required. Most of the recent advances pertain to the statistical properties of the SFA and DEA procedures. Future efforts need to concentrate on developing coherent theoretical frameworks for the analysis of efficiency that will better inform model construction, noting that the appropriate theoretical basis may depend on the purpose of analysis. Allied to this is the requirement for greater consideration of the output/objective weights to be applied when, as is usual, organizations produce multiple outputs or pursue multiple objectives, or when the objective functions of regulators and organizations differ. In such circumstances, rather than collapsing multiple objectives into a single measure of performance and labelling shortfalls in performance as inefficiency, it may be more fruitful to undertake simultaneous analysis of multiple objectives. This would allow greater flexibility in modelling the production process and provide more relevant information to induce desirable changes in behaviour.

REFERENCES

Aigner, D., Lovell, C.A.K. and Schmidt, P. (1977) Formulation and estimation of stochastic frontier production function models, *Journal of Econometrics,* 6: 21–37.

Allen, R., Athanassopoulos, A., Dyson, R.G. and Thanassoulis, E. (1997) Weight restrictions and value judgements in data envelopment analysis: evolution, development and future directions, *Annals of Operations Research,* 73: 13–34.

Bagust, A., Place, M. and Posnett, J.W. (1999) Dynamics of bed use in accommodating emergency admissions: stochastic simulation model, *British Medical Journal,* 319: 155–8.

Bailey, T.C. and Hewson, P.J. (forthcoming) Simultaneous modelling of multiple traffic safety performance indicators using a multivariate generalized linear mixed model, *Journal of the Royal Statistical Society,* Series A.

Banker, R.D., Charnes, A. and Cooper, W.W. (1984) Some models for estimating technical and scale inefficiencies in data envelopment analysis, *Management Science,* 30: 1078–92.

Battese, G.E. and Coelli, T.J. (1988) Prediction of firm-level technical efficiencies with a generalized frontier production function and panel data, *Journal of Econometrics,* 38: 387–99.

Breyer, F. (1987) On the specification of a hospital cost function, *Journal of Health Economics,* 6: 147–57.

Browne, W.J. and Rasbash, J. (2001) Multilevel modelling, in A. Bryman and M. Hardy (eds) *Handbook of Data Analysis.* London: Sage.

Charnes, A., Cooper, W.W. and Rhodes, E. (1978) Measuring the efficiency of decision-making units, *European Journal of Operational Research,* 2: 429–44.

Charnes, A., Cooper, W.W., Lewin, A.Y. and Seiford, L.M. (1994) *Data Envelopment Analysis: Theory, Methodology and Applications.* Boston, MA: Kluwer Academic.

Coelli, T. and Perelman, S. (1996) *Efficiency Measurement, Multiple-output Technologies and Distance Functions: With Application to European Railways.* CREPP Discussion Paper No. 96/05. University of Liege: Liege, Belgium.

Coelli, T., Prasada Rao, D.S. and Battese, G.E. (1998) *An Introduction to Efficiency and Productivity Analysis.* Boston, MA: Kluwer Academic.

Cornwell, C., Schmidt, P. and Sickles, R. (1990) Production frontiers with cross-sectional and time-series variation in efficiency levels, *Journal of Econometrics,* 46: 185–200.

Dopuch, N. and Gupta, M. (1997) Estimation of benchmark performance standards: an application to public school expenditures, *Journal of Accounting and Economics,* 23: 147–61.

Dor, A. (1994) Non-minimum cost functions and the stochastic frontier: on applications to health care providers, *Journal of Health Economics,* 13: 329–34.

Dyson, R.G. and Thanassoulis, E. (1988) Reducing weight flexibility in data envelopment analysis, *Journal of the Operational Research Society,* 39(6): 563–76.

Ellis, R.P. (1998) Creaming, skimping, and dumping: provider competition on the intensive and extensive margins, *Journal of Health Economics,* 17: 537–55.

Farrell, M.J. (1957) The measurement of productive efficiency, *Journal of the Royal Statistical Society,* Series A, 120(3): 253–90.

Farsi, M., Filippini, M. and Kuenzle, M. (2003) Unobserved heterogeneity in stochastic cost frontier models, 8th European Workshop on Efficiency and Productivity Analysis Oviedo, Spain.

Fernández, J.L. and Forder, J. (2002) *Unblocking Hospital Beds: the role of Social Care, PSSRU, LSE Health and Social Care.* London: London School of Economics.

Folland, S. and Hofler, R. (2001) How reliable are hospital efficiency estimates? Exploiting the dual to homothetic production, *Health Economics,* 10: 683–98.

Giuffrida, A. and Gravelle, H. (2001) Measuring performance in primary care: econometric analysis and DEA, *Applied Economics,* 33: 163–75.

Giuffrida, A., Gravelle, H. and Sutton, M. (2000) Efficiency and administrative costs in primary care, *Journal of Health Economics,* 19: 983–1006.

Greene, W.H. (1993) The econometric approach to efficiency analysis, in H.O. Fried, C.A.K. Lovell and S.S. Schmidt (eds) *The Measurement of Productive Efficiency: Techniques and Applications.* New York: Oxford University Press.

Greene, W.H. (forthcoming) Distinguishing between heterogeneity and inefficiency: stochastic frontier analysis of the World Health Organisation's panel data on national health care systems, *Health Economics.*

Hadley, J. and Zuckerman, S. (1994) The role of efficiency measurement in hospital rate setting, *Journal of Health Economics,* 13: 335–40.

Hauck, K. and Street, A. (2004) *Performance Assessment in the Context of Multiple Objectives: A Multivariate Multilevel Analysis* (mimeo). York: Centre for Health Economics (CHE), University of York.

Hausman, J. (1978) Specification tests in econometrics, *Econometrica,* 46: 1251–71.

Hollingsworth, B., Dawson, P.J. and Maniadakis, N. (1999) Efficiency measurement of health care: a review of non-parametric methods and applications, *Health Care Management Science,* 2(3): 161–72.

Horrace, W.C. and Schmidt, P. (1996) Confidence statements for efficiency estimates from stochastic frontier models, *Journal of Productivity Analysis,* 7: 257–82.

Jacobs, R. (2001) Alternative methods to examine hospital efficiency: data envelopment analysis and stochastic frontier analysis, *Health Care Management Science,* 4(2): 103–16.

Jensen, U. (2000) Is it efficient to analyse efficiency rankings? *Empirical Economics,* 25: 189–208.

Joskow, P.L. (1980) The effects of competition and regulation on hospital bed supply and reservation quality of the hospital, *The Bell Journal of Economics,* 11: 421–47.

Kooreman, P. (1994a) Nursing home care in the Netherlands: a nonparametric efficiency analysis, *Journal of Health Economics,* 13: 301–16.

Kooreman, P. (1994b) Data envelopment analysis and parametric frontier estimation: complementary tools, *Journal of Health Economics,* 13: 345–6.

Kumbhakar, S.C. (1990) Production frontiers, panel data, and time-varying technical inefficiency, *Journal of Econometrics,* 46: 201–11.

Kumbhakar, S.C. and Lovell, C.A.K. (2000) *Stochastic Frontier Analysis.* New York: Cambridge University Press.

Linna, M. (1998) Measuring hospital cost efficiency with panel data models, *Health Economics,* 7: 415–27.

Maniadakis, N., Hollingsworth, B. and Thanassoulis, E. (1999) The impact of the internal market on hospital efficiency, productivity and service quality, *Health Care Management Science,* 2: 75–85.

Morrison, P.C.J., Johnston, W.E. and Frengley, G.A.G. (2000) Efficiency in New Zealand sheep and beef farming: the impacts of regulatory reform, *Review of Economics and Statistics,* 82: 325–37.

Newhouse, J.P. (1994) Frontier estimation: how useful a tool for health economics? *Journal of Health Economics,* 13: 317–22.

Nutley, S. and Smith, P.C. (1998) League tables for performance improvement in health care, *Journal of Health Services Research and Policy,* 3(1): 50–7.

Office of Water Trading (1999) *Future Water and Sewerage Charges 2000–05: Draft Determination.* London: OFWAT.

Pedraja-Chaparro, F., Salinas-Jiménez, J. and Smith, P. (1997) On the role of weight restrictions in data envelopment analysis, *Journal of Productivity Analysis,* 8(2): 215–30.

Pitt, M. and Lee, L. (1981) The measurement and sources of technical inefficiency in Indonesian weaving industry, *Journal of Development Economics,* 9: 43–64.

Public Services Productivity Panel (2004) Press notice 4. London: UK Treasury.

Puig-Junoy, J. (1998) Technical efficiency in the clinical management of critically ill patients, *Health Economics,* 7: 263–77.

Rice, N. and Jones, A. (1997) Multilevel models and health economics, *Health Economics,* 6: 561–75.

Roll, Y., Cook, W. and Golany, B. (1991) Controlling factor weights in data envelopment analysis, *IIE Transactions,* 23(1): 2–9.

Schleifer, A. (1985) A theory of yardstick competition, *Rand Journal of Economics,* 16: 319–27.

Schmidt, P. (1985) Frontier production functions, *Econometric Reviews,* 4: 289–328.

Schmidt, P. and Lin, T. (1984) Simple tests of alternative specifications in stochastic frontier models, *Journal of Econometrics,* 24: 349–61.

Schmidt, P. and Sickles, R.C. (1984) Production frontiers and panel data, *Journal of Business and Economic Statistics,* 2(4): 367–74.

Simar, L. and Wilson, P.W. (2002) Estimation and inference in two-stage, semi-parametric models of production processes. Paper presented at Workshop on Quantitative Methods for the Measurement of Organizational Efficiency, Institute for Fiscal Studies, University College London.

Skinner, J. (1994) What do stochastic frontier cost functions tell us about inefficiency? *Journal of Health Economics,* 13: 323–8.

Smith, P. (1998) *Data Envelopment Analysis in Health Care: An Introductory Note.* York: Centre for Health Economics (CHE). University of York.

Stigler, G. (1976) The Xistence of X-efficiency, *American Economic Review,* 66: 213–16.

Street, A. (2003) How much confidence should we place in efficiency estimates? *Health Economics,* 12: 895–907.

Thanassoulis, E. (1993) A comparison of regression analysis and data envelopment analysis as alternative methods for performance assessments, *Journal of the Operational Research Society,* 44(11): 1129–44.

Thompson, R.G., Langemeier, L.N., Lee, C.T. and Thrall, R.M. (1990) The role of multiplier bounds in efficiency analysis with application to Kansas farming, *Journal of Econometrics,* 46(1/2): 93–108.

Timmer, C.P. (1971) Using a probabilistic frontier production function to measure technical efficiency, *Journal of Political Economy,* 79: 776–94.

Tulkens, H. (1993) On FDH efficiency analysis: some methodological issues and applications to retail banking, courts and urban transit, *Journal of Productivity Analysis,* 4: 183–210.

Vitaliano, D.F. and Toren, M. (1994a) Cost and efficiency in nursing homes: a stochastic frontier approach, *Journal of Health Economics,* 13: 281–300.

Vitaliano, D.F. and Toren, M. (1994b) Frontier analysis: a reply to Skinner, Dor and Newhouse, *Journal of Health Economics,* 13: 341–3.

Wagstaff, A. (1989) Estimating efficiency in the hospital sector: a comparison of three statistical cost frontier models, *Applied Economics,* 21: 659–72.

Wong, Y.H.B. and Beasley, J.E. (1990) Restricting weight flexibility in data envelopment analysis, *Journal of the Operational Research Society,* 41(9): 829–35.

Zuckerman, S., Hadley, J. and Iezzoni, L. (1994) Measuring hospital efficiency with frontier cost functions, *Journal of Health Economics,* 13: 255–80.

7

INCENTIVES AND THE UK MEDICAL LABOUR MARKET
Karen Bloor and Alan Maynard

INTRODUCTION

All health care systems are labour intensive. While nurses are the largest single component of expenditure, doctors, and the decisions made and actions taken by them, are the most powerful determinant of health expenditure and activity. UK physician workforce planners since before the existence of the National Health Service (NHS) have estimated the required numbers of physicians using physician/population ratios. This approach appears to imply that labour force activity and patient outcomes can only be changed by proportionate increases in all inputs. This limits the potential to make any changes without the substantial time lag of training more medical staff. It also neglects the role of incentive systems, both financial (e.g. payment methods) and non-financial (e.g. regulation) in influencing activity rates. There may be potential for improving the productivity of this workforce – for example, by changing reward systems and incentive structures, or by better regulation and management, ideally managing both process and outcomes.

This chapter considers the economic literature relating to the effect these factors have on productivity. The first section looks at the economics literature on doctor behaviour. The second considers methods to monitor clinical performance, while the third looks at the reform of doctors' contracts in the UK health service between 2000 and 2004. Finally, the fourth section offers some conclusions.

ECONOMIC MODELS OF DOCTOR BEHAVIOUR

Doctors as agents

The sub-discipline of health economics is largely concerned with institutional and organizational responses to market failures, in particular responses to a situation of pervasive uncertainty:

> When there is uncertainty, information or knowledge becomes a commodity ... The value of information is frequently not known in any meaningful sense to the buyer; if, indeed, he knew enough to measure the value of information, he would know the information itself. But information, in the form of skilled care, is precisely what is being bought from most physicians.
>
> (Arrow 1963: 946)

Because of information asymmetry, patient and doctor initiate an agency relationship, with the doctor helping the patient to make choices. If the agency relationship was perfect, or 'complete', the doctor would take on the patient's point of view in its entirety, acting as if he or she were the patient – all choices would be made to maximize the patient's well-being (Evans 1984). However, the agency relationship between doctor and patient is not perfect. Doctors have interests of their own – 'income, leisure, professional satisfaction, which are partially congruent and partly in conflict with that of the patient' (Evans 1984: 75). An additional complication is that the patient may be unable to judge the performance of the doctor before, or even after, an intervention, which limits the potential of perform-ance-related pay as a response to incomplete agency. Professionalism and self-regulation have therefore emerged, with codes of medical ethics and conduct developed to reassure the consumer that the doc-tor will act as the patient's 'agent' and in the consumer's best interests.

Alongside the imperfect agency relationship between doctor and patient, hospital specialists, as they often control the actions of teams of staff and, by their actions, control substantial budgets, must act as agents of their employers – hospitals, or health service funders such as government. Doctors can, therefore, be viewed as 'double agents' (Blomqvist 1991).

Doctors and incentives

Despite the complexity and incompleteness of the agency relationship in determining incentives, traditional utilitarian theories still have a role in predicting physician behaviour. Those defining economic models have tended to focus on explicit financial incentives, and particularly on payment mechanisms.

The method of payment of providers in the health care system can have an impact on their behaviour and, therefore, on the achievement of the objectives of the health care system (efficiency, equity, cost containment). The central economic problem inherent in devising a payment system is the provision of efficient incentives to promote appropriate behaviour, and to allow stated objectives to be pursued. One major difficulty with devising an incentive-compatible contract in this agency relationship is that of measuring performance. Health outcomes are problematic to measure and may not be directly attributable to the performance of the individual health care provider, but rather to a team, or to other determinants of health status. In addition, attempts to derive an incentive-compatible contract focus exclusively on efficiency goals. Cost containment and (particularly) equity goals have not been incorporated into this area of economic analysis. Orientating reform towards equity goals as well as efficiency goals creates a substantial challenge, and may require policy instruments other than payment reform.

Explicit incentives: payment mechanisms and financial incentives

Standard labour economic analysis of payment systems suggests that firms manipulate the level and structure of wages to induce workers to supply the desired quantity and quality of labour (Elliott 1991). Two main pay structures are used, representing the extremes of a continuum: time rates, where workers are paid for each hour of time they spend at work; and piece rates, where pay is related directly to output. In practice, firms often combine these methods. Where health care is concerned, these translate to salary (time rates) and fee-for-service (FFS) (piece rates), and capitation forms an intermediate method.

The three main methods of paying doctors and other health care professionals – FFS, capitation and salary (see Table 7.1) – are, in practice, often mixed (Robinson 1999). For example, general practitioners (GPs – family doctors) in the UK have traditionally received a basic practice allowance (essentially a salary component), a capitation fee for each patient, and also some fees per item of service for targeted interventions. However, nearly 40 per cent of GPs are now salaried. Similarly, in US-managed care organizations, various blended forms of reimbursement are used to pay doctors, even when

Table 7.1 Doctor payment systems

Payment type	Definition	Incentive effects				
		Incentive to increase activity	Incentive to decrease activity	Incentive to shift patients' costs to others	Incentive to target the poor	Controls cost of doctor employment
Fee-for-service (FFS)	Payment for each medical act	Yes	No	No	Maybe*	No
Salary	Payment per unit of time input (e.g. per month)	No	Yes	Yes	No	Yes
Capitation	Payment per patient for care within a given time period (e.g. a year)	No	Yes	Yes	Maybe*	Yes

* If FFS payments for treating poor patients exceed those for treating the middle classes, or if capitation fees are adequately weighted.

the health care plans are paid on a straightforward capitation basis (Robinson 1999).

The main focus of economic analysis of the agency relationship in health care, particularly under FFS payment systems, has been to address the existence of supplier-induced demand (SID) (Evans 1984; McGuire 2000). The dual input into the provider's utility function, including both patient health and provider income, creates potential incentives for over-treatment, with doctors able to generate substantial demand and subvert the way markets normally function (Folland *et al.* 1993). SID may be the product either of a desire to maximize income or pursue a target income (subject to work-leisure trade-offs), or of a desire to do more and reduce uncertainty in the processes of diagnosing and treating illness. Doctors tend to assume that more means better and their desire to do their best for the patient may lead to increased activity. Distinguishing between the effects of these two possible motives is not easy.

An FFS payment system contains explicit incentives to increase activity. It provides an effective incentive for physicians to see many patients and perform difficult procedures (Robinson 1999). However, this activity is not necessarily efficient, and may be fragmented, so the incentive system can limit the achievement of cost containment and efficiency objectives. Unnecessary activity is stimulated under an FFS system, and relies on implicit incentives – for example, self-regulation and medical ethics, to limit harm. Fee systems also marginalize that which is not incentivized, and for which no fee is attached.

Capitation payment does not contain incentives to over-treat, which are present within FFS payment systems. There is some incentive to maintain quality of care and therefore attract and retain patients, but this is limited by information problems. There may also be incentives to undertake health promotion and preventative care, as this may reduce costs later in the health care process. Capitation may create, particularly if patients are ill-informed, undesirable incentives for physicians to err on the side of withholding potentially beneficial treatment (Blomqvist 1991), and also provides incentives for frequent referral to other clinicians (Robinson 1999) and for cost shifting – for example, from primary to secondary care. In addition it may, particularly if the payment is not adjusted accurately to reflect the epidemiological risk of the population, reward physicians who attract a relatively healthy patient mix and penalize those who care for the chronically ill, causing doctors to avoid such costly patients (Newhouse 1996; Robinson 1999; McGuire 2000).

Salary payments do not contain incentives to over-treat, so maintain cost control, but they may contain incentives to withhold care, or to shift costs. Salary payment systems (time rates) are, therefore, opposite to FFS systems (piece rates) in terms of incentive structures. If salary is used without any supplementary explicit incentives (such as bonus payments), regulation or implicit incentive structures may be required to increase activity rates.

To avoid the limitations of any of the three individual payment methods, blended systems are increasingly used, supplemented by bonus or target payments. Although mixed payment systems have appeal, it may be that the more sophisticated and complex the pay system, the greater the scope for 'gaming' such systems, as this behaviour is increasingly difficult to monitor.

Explicit incentives: bonus payments and performance-related pay

Economic models of the agency relationship emphasize the need for an incentive-compatible contract between principal and agent, generally incorporating some form of performance-related pay. In health care this is less than straightforward as, although there is an agency relationship between doctor and patient in an individual consultation, the employer of the doctor is not the patient but a third party (most often government in publicly-provided systems like the UK NHS). Nevertheless, a government White Paper in 1999 (Cabinet Office 1999) outlined the intention to 'modernize' and 'incentivize' government employees, encouraging the use of performance-related pay schemes.

Some bonus pay exists for UK doctors. Hospital specialists are eligible to receive distinction awards, which aim to reward 'excellence'. GPs are also paid bonus payments for reaching target levels of, for example, immunization and screening, and other income-based incentives have been used, particularly since 1990 (Whynes and Baines 1998).

Burgess and Metcalfe (1999) investigated the use of incentive schemes in the public and private sectors in Britain, using a cross-sectional survey of workplaces to compare types of pay system used. Their findings confirmed that incentive pay systems are far less widespread in the public sector than the private sector, and that performance-related pay tends to be used when measuring output is easy, with systems of merit pay used when measuring output is difficult. This conclusion is supported in relation to reward of UK hospital specialists: the only form of explicit incentive pay is the system of discretionary points and distinction awards, which rewards vaguely defined 'excellence' and is based on subjective assessment of 'merit' or 'distinction' rather than objective measurement of work activity and patient outcomes.

Implicit incentives

Economic theory using models of explicit financial incentives alone is not an accurate predictor of the behaviour of doctors. For example, econometric analyses based on financial incentives alone have been able to explain less than 10 per cent of observable variation in the hours worked by US doctors (Reinhardt 1999). Choice of method of payment alone is but a partial account: 'Casual empiricism tells us that there is more to incentives than simply more jam today. Many individuals who do not receive any performance related bonus are nevertheless strongly motivated by the possibility of either promotion within the organisation or a better job offer from an outside firm' (Burgess and Metcalfe 1999: 24).

Thus individuals, even those interested solely in financial gain, are not simply interested in their current rewards, but are also motivated to increase effort by the likelihood of future rewards over a lifetime, or 'career concerns' (Holmstrom 1982a, 1982b; Dewatripont *et al.* 1999a, 1999b). Wages depend on expected productivity, which is a function of observed performance in previous periods. This creates an 'implicit contract', linking current performance to future wages (Holmstrom 1982a, 1982b; Burgess and Metcalfe 1999). Dewatripont *et al.* (1999a, 1999b) suggest that incentives generated through career concerns may be particularly important in the public sector. Their findings suggest that changing organizational design could improve performance in the public sector: improving clarity of goals and minimizing the number of tasks to each official may improve incentive structures through their career concerns (Burgess and Metcalfe 1999; Dewatripont *et al.* 1999a, 1999b). However, empirical evidence testing the predictions of models of career concerns is minimal and contradictory in private sector workers, and non-existent in government officials (Burgess and Metcalfe 1999).

Applying implicit incentive or career concern models to the reward of UK doctors, and the link between reward and activity, is not straightforward. First, the conditions for successful government agencies (Wilson 1989; Dewatripont *et al.* 1999a, 1999b) are not obvious in the UK NHS. Goals of the health service, at local hospital level, are vague and often unclear, and doctors undertake a variety of tasks, not just treatment of patients. UK hospital specialists have no obvious promotion structure: once fully trained, and in a 'consultant' post, hospital doctors are essentially at the top of their careers. Without taking on additional responsibilities (such as management or administration) the only reward systems for specialists are discretionary points and distinction awards: merit pay rather than promotion. In terms of signals to current and future employers, or those allocating discretionary points and distinction awards, increasing activity in terms of treating NHS patients may be only a weak signal of work effort, as employers (chief executives of NHS Trusts) typically do not engage in monitoring activity rates of hospital consultants, and activity rates are not generally used to allocate distinction awards.

For career concerns to improve motivation and increase NHS activity, signals of activity of hospital specialists to hospital managers, and those allocating further awards, have to be clear. Other work undertaken by hospital specialists (e.g. teaching, research, Royal College activity) may be a more obvious signal to employers and medical peers (who determine distinction awards), and may be more of a 'career concern' to UK hospital doctors.

The situation is similar for GPs: once they are appointed a GP principal, and partner in their practice, there is no real option for further promotion, so 'career concerns' are minimal. This may explain the explicit nature of the incentives incorporated into the new GP contract. Without total reform of the GP contract, the potential of implicit incentives to influence activity rates is very limited.

Even with implicit incentives, career concern models of employee behaviour still imply that financial incentives determine behaviour: the timescale is simply longer, and behaviour now determines income later. This still represents an oversimplification, particularly in medicine, as non-financial incentives (such as trust, duty, altruism and reputation) are extremely important in determining behaviour (Maynard and Bloor 2003).

Non-financial incentives may take a variety of forms. In medicine, a sense of 'duty' is strongly reinforced by professional codes and self-regulation. In addition, funders of health care, insurers and/or government inevitably regulate the medical profession through contracts and other mechanisms, including licensing systems. Economists have viewed medicine as a 'reputation good' – a good for which consumers rely on the information provided by friends, neighbours and others to select from the various services available (Folland *et al.* 1993). Providers of health care also respond to asymmetry of information by professionalism and licensure, where systems of self-regulation are introduced as an indicator of reputation (Evans 1984). Until relatively recently, licensure and self-regulation have been the main restraint on the activity of the medical profession. However, self-regulation relies on the *trust* of patients and employers. O'Neill (2002) refers to a 'crisis of trust' in recent years, with a consequent (and sometimes perverse) 'accountability revolution'. This includes the introduction of job plans and appraisal for hospital doctors, reflecting an erosion of trust between employers and physicians, and also increased regulation through the General Medical Council (2000), and through new institutions such as the National Institute for Clinical Excellence (NICE) (Department of Health 1999) and the Commission for Health Improvement (2003).

Summary: economics and reward and activity of doctors

Economic concepts contribute substantially to debate about reward and activity of NHS doctors. Current NHS hospital payment systems are all based on salary, which, as discussed, contains no incentives for individual activity. The bonus payments that currently reward hospital specialists (discretionary points and distinction awards) are merit pay, and are largely unrelated to the rates of NHS activity of individual consultants. In primary care, capitation payment in principle should make doctors responsive to patient demands, as they wish to recruit patients to, and retain them on, their 'lists'. However, in practice, patients rarely switch GPs and GPs often have no wish to increase their list size, so responsiveness is limited.

Economists accept that short-term financial incentives are not the only determinant of employee behaviour. Implicit incentives or 'career concerns' models incorporate a longer-term aspect to incentive structures, recognizing that individuals are motivated by long-term income, based on promotion and other career structures. Career concerns may differ with the age of the doctor, and the stage of career reached. However, opportunities for promotion are limited for hospital consultants and for GP principals. For career concerns to improve motivation and increase activity, signals of activity have to be clear, and long-term incentives present. At present, non-clinical work may be more of a 'career concern' to hospital specialists. It is difficult to assess the career concerns faced by UK GPs, which may help to explain recurring 'crises' in the morale, recruitment and retention of GPs. More broadly, economists since Adam Smith have recognized that doctors, like other citizens, are motivated not only by financial rewards (short- or long-term) but also by reputation and other non-financial incentives (Smith 1790).

The interweaving effects of explicit incentives (immediate financial rewards) and implicit incentives (long-term reward, and non-financial issues such as reputation) make the design and evaluation of reward systems for doctors a complex task. While predictions for each financial payment system can be made, observation of the effects of these explicit incentives may be difficult because of countervailing or complementary effects from implicit, non-financial incentives such as duty, trust and self-regulation. It is necessary to balance explicit financial incentives and implicit non-financial incentives to meet policy objectives, such as increasing activity and improved patient outcomes in a cost-effective manner with minimum necessary transaction costs.

CLINICAL PERFORMANCE

In most manufacturing and service industries, the relationship between inputs (staff time, raw materials) and outputs (goods or services provided) is a key indicator of success or failure. But in UK health care, this productivity relationship is almost totally neglected.

In health care, monitoring productivity would ideally mean measuring 'health' produced as a result of inputs into health care, particularly staff time but also other resource inputs. It is difficult to measure 'health improvements' at an individual or population level, and health status measures such as EQ-5D (Kind *et al.* 1998) are not yet used to measure population health over time. Furthermore, health outcomes are a product of many factors, not just health care (McKeown 1976; Acheson 1998). As it is so difficult to measure 'health' and attribute changes to the health care system, proxy measures of output or activity are often used.

Hospital activity rates

For decades, the NHS has routinely collected hospital activity data, but this has not been used in planning, policymaking or management. Exploring trends in activity over time, data show a consistent increase in the number of discharges and deaths or finished consultant episodes (FCEs) in the UK hospital sector (Office of Health Economics 2003). However, this is mostly explained by increases in the number of staff working in that sector. Episodes per doctor have actually decreased over time, from 258 discharges and deaths in 1951 to 198 FCEs in 2001/2 (see Figure 7.1).

Time series data make no adjustment for severity of patient case mix, 'quality' of patient care or health outcome. Clinicians may be handling fewer cases but their complexity may have increased (as less serious patients remain outside hospital) and their health outcomes may have improved.

Attempts have been made to measure activity and productivity over time, particularly using the Hospital and Community Health Services (HCHS) 'cost weighted activity index' (CWAI), and the 'labour productivity index'. Both use national average reference costs as a proxy for case-mix adjustment, which facilitates comparisons between Trusts, but such comparisons have been criticized due to the exclusion of non-clinical activity, the inaccuracy of the cost weights and the neglect of subcontracted staff (Appleby 1996).

In addition to attempts to measure activity over time, there has been some cross-sectional measurement of variations in consultant activity in the UK, particularly by Yates and colleagues (Yates 1995), using routine NHS data such as Hospital Episode Statistics and unpublished government reports. These data have been analysed in some detail in surgical procedures in the West Midlands' region of England, revealing large variations in clinical practice in both emergency and elective procedures, which could not be accounted for adequately by differences in case mix, or teaching and research commitments (Yates 1995).

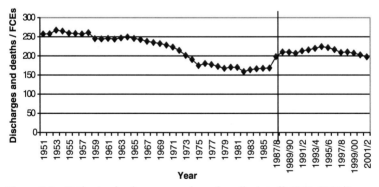

Figure 7.1 Patient episodes per member of medical staff, 1951–2001/2
Note: Change in definition in 1988 from discharges and deaths to finished consultant episodes (FCEs).
Source: Office of Health Economics (2003).

Table 7.2 Activity rates of hospital specialists (finished consultant episodes per year)

	Number of specialists	Mean activity	SD	Quartiles			Interquartile variation
				25	50	75	
General surgery	1223	1139	548	779	1126	1443	1.85
Urology	410	1129	509	936	1290	1730	1.85
Trauma & orthopaedics	1136	668	268	504	663	809	1.60
ENT	462	824	405	603	779	1022	1.69
Ophthalmology	604	643	337	439	611	799	1.82

Table 7.3 Case-mix adjusted activity (£000 activity per year)

	Number of consultants	Mean	SD	Quartiles			Interquartile variation
				25	50	75	
General surgery	1223	1013	435	762	1010	1270	1.67
Urology	410	825	371	578	814	1037	1.80
Trauma & orthopaedics	1136	974	391	742	971	1190	1.60
ENT	462	545	255	404	527	677	1.68
Ophthalmology	604	388	196	269	370	475	1.77

A simple distribution of activity per consultant in five surgical specialities shows considerable variation. Tables 7.2 and 7.3 describe consultant activity rates in each of five surgical specialties in 1998/9, using episodes with and without case-mix adjustment. The tables show considerable variation between consultants. Interquartile variation is around 1.6–1.85, which shows that the top 25 per cent of consultants have activity rates 60 to 85 per cent higher than the bottom 25 per cent. Using case-mix-adjusted data, interquartile variation remains at 1.6 to 1.8. Figures 7.2 and 7.3 illustrate consultant activity rates for one of the five specialties (general surgery).

The variation observed may be the product of imperfect data, particularly the medical workforce census (which has some limitations), or due to public sector bottlenecks such as hospitals hiring medical staff in numbers exceeding their capacity to provide theatre and other complementary resources. It could also relate to consultant behaviour – for example, in terms of private practice, although part-time surgical consultants in the NHS appear to have higher activity levels than those of full-time practitioners (Bloor *et al.* 2004). This variation in activity is consistent with wider academic literature on medical practice variations, which have proved persistent across different health care systems and over time (McPherson *et al.* 1982; Andersen and Mooney 1990).

How such variations in activity relate to variations in patient care and outcomes is unclear. Specialization in surgical areas such as vascular and upper gastrointestinal diseases is associated with better outcomes (NHS Centre for Reviews and Dissemination 1996). Recent US research shows that variations in expenditure (in Medicare) are due to volume effects: residents in high spending regions received 60 per cent more care 'but did not have lower mortality rates, better functional status or higher satisfaction' (Fisher *et al.* 2003: 289). This work demonstrates the necessity to link analysis of activity variations with outcomes, even if this is restricted initially to mortality or other crude indicators. Hopefully increasing analysis of practice variation in the NHS will precipitate clinical and managerial interest in such relationships, thereby hastening the collection of improved outcome data.

Activity rates in general practice

Activity measures, limited in NHS hospital care, are practically non-existent in primary care. The UK model of general practice, well established, and generally advocated as 'efficient', is essentially a

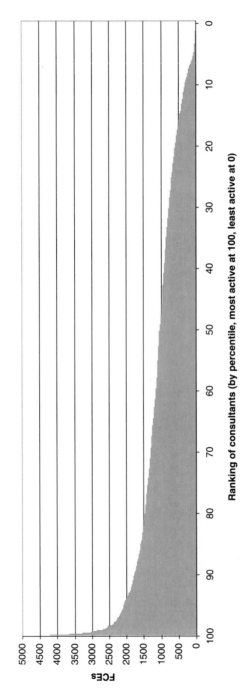

Figure 7.2 Ranked activity per consultant surgeon: general surgery, finished consultant episodes per year, 1999–2000 data

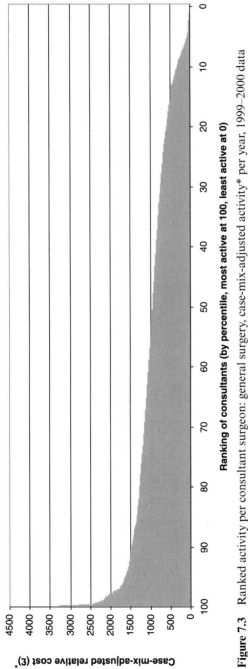
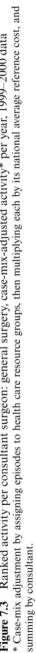

Figure 7.3 Ranked activity per consultant surgeon: general surgery, case-mix-adjusted activity* per year, 1999–2000 data
* Case-mix adjustment by assigning episodes to health care resource groups, then multiplying each by its national average reference cost, and summing by consultant.

black box in terms of data and information systems that facilitate comparisons. While UK NHS hospital physicians are salaried employees, their general practitioner colleagues are self-employed with (until recent reforms) a contract of remarkable vagueness, and are barely monitored.

There is no national system of data collection for primary care activity. Sources of information on primary care rely on the annual General Household Survey and periodic National Morbidity surveys. As a consequence of this limited investment in data collection, all too little is known about many aspects of the primary care system.

The number of GPs in the UK has increased steadily over recent decades. GP principals have increased from around 20,000 in 1951 (40 per 100,000 population) to 34,500 in 2002 (58 per 100,000 population). This has meant that patient list sizes have fallen continuously over time, from 2500 patients per UK GP in 1951 to 1582 in 2002 (Office of Health Economics 2003). In addition, and particularly since the 1991 reforms and the introduction of GP fundholding, non-GP staff have been increasingly employed in GP practices. Overall, consultations have increased gradually over time, but consultations per GP have remained relatively stable since 1975, at between 8000 and 9000 per year (see Figure 7.4).

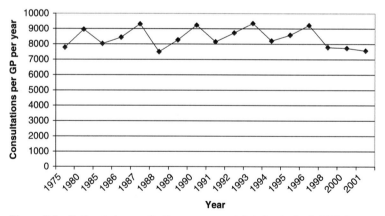

Figure 7.4   Estimated consultations per unrestricted principal, UK, by age group
Source: Office of Health Economics (2003).

CURRENT REFORM OF MEDICAL CONTRACTS

'The unnerving discovery every Minister of Health makes at or near the outset of his term of office is that the only subject he is ever destined to discuss with the medical profession is money' (Powell 1966: 14).

The period between 2000 and 2004 was one of renegotiation of the contracts of employment for both GPs and hospital specialists, with systems changing in the most radical way since 1948. The objective of these reforms was to ensure recruitment and retention in the profession, and also to increase NHS activity and deliver the 'modernization' agenda by using FFS complements to existing contracts. The latter will require detailed performance management by the profession and managers. Any change in contract terms and conditions is likely to create gainers and losers, and human nature ensures that those who gain keep quiet, whereas those who potentially could lose create resistance and conflict. Contract reform, always controversial, requires compensation of losers as well as an increase in the remuneration of those who gain, resulting in substantial costs for any change.

The contract for hospital medical specialists

Methods and levels of reimbursement of medical specialists ('consultants') have been a matter of intense policy debate for many decades. Attempts to reform consultant contracts have historically been met with substantial resistance. The Labour governments elected in 1997 and 2001 optimistically hoped to overcome the problems of the past, but also encountered similar resistance.

The NHS Plan (Department of Health 2000) expressed the government's aim of a fundamental overhaul of the national contract for UK hospital specialists, 'to reward and incentivize those who do most for the NHS' (p. 79). Proposals for achieving this were initially published in February 2001 (Department of Health 2001a, 2001b), influenced by the view that private medical practice reduced NHS productivity. It was proposed that newly-appointed NHS consultants would be obliged to serve a period of seven years working exclusively in the NHS. In addition to this, career payment scales were related to NHS activity and the possibility of considerable enhancements in pay. However, both junior doctors and specialists were opposed to enhanced control of their public-private time allocations and 'management interference' in their autonomy.

A revised framework for the contract was eventually published by the Department of Health in June 2002 (Department of Health & BMA Central Consultants and Specialists Committee 2002). This eliminated the seven-year indenture clause but was accompanied by indications of an intention to manage practice in a more detailed way. It also required practitioners to agree that the NHS had a first call on any overtime, with established consultants having to offer the NHS four hours and new consultants eight hours per week before they could undertake private practice.

The new contract was accepted in Scotland and Northern Ireland but a large majority of English and Welsh consultants rejected it. The Secretary of State refused further negotiation and published new proposals (Department of Health 2003). Where there was support for the published contract framework, Trusts and consultants were encouraged to implement it. Elsewhere, Trusts and Primary Care Trusts (PCTs) were asked to introduce a new system of annual incentives, 'to reward consultants who achieve the most for NHS patients' (Department of Health 2003). Local incentive schemes were encouraged, with payments to consultants in the form of annual non-recurrent bonuses, based on 'objective measures of performance' in relation to NHS modernization targets. Examples of incentive schemes suggested by the Department of Health included a financial reward to consultants or teams who exceeded a benchmark level of case-mix-adjusted activity (e.g. a regional or national median), linking the reward to the amount of activity and using data similar to that illustrated in Figure 7.3 to provide an FFS supplement to NHS salaries. This reflected a belief, partly based on variations illustrated by Yates (1995) and Bloor *et al.* (2004), that spare capacity existed and could be exploited.

In July 2003 a new Secretary of State compromised, and achieved agreement with the British Medical Association (BMA) consultant negotiators. The obligatory NHS overtime commitment was reduced to four hours for all consultants, the obligation to carry out evening and weekend work was removed, out-of-hours sessions were reduced to three hours, and some additional holiday allowance was introduced. Now that the contract has been accepted by the consultant body, the proposed FFS package appears to be redundant.

Given variations in surgical activity as seen in the Hospital Episode Statistics (HES) data (see Figures 7.2 and 7.3, and Bloor *et al.* (2004)), there is considerable scope to augment activity by shifting the mean and increasing practitioner activity. Whether this is better done by FFS, target payments and/or more active management of workload and activity is an empirical matter. There is a risk that none of these instruments will be acceptable to the profession. Consequently, it is essential to evaluate any reforms so that future policy choices are informed and cost effectiveness ensured.

The 2003 consultant contract demonstrates that, temporarily at least, the demand for clinical autonomy (defined as the absence of detailed and effective local management of activity and outcomes) has triumphed. At the same time, the personal income of consultants has been substantially enhanced – basic salaries have been considerably increased, and distinction awards remain (repackaged and renamed but with very little significant change). This BMA 'victory' should ensure that hospital specialists do not disrupt the NHS modernization plans. The new contract offers no effective management of the large variations in activity, which may indicate under-utilization of NHS capacity.

More vigorous and systematic local management of clinicians is inevitable as the new NHS pricing system (Department of Health 2004) and Foundation Hospitals (Department of Health 2002) are developed. Also, hopefully, re-accreditation of clinicians by the General Medical Council (GMC) will focus on comparative activity and outcome rates. To better regulate clinical practice and the performance of doctors and other health professionals, better measures of patient outcome and patient case mix are essential, along with development of measures to address practice variations. In the short term, outcomes are measured in terms of mortality and perhaps readmission rates, and case-mix adjusters are imperfect.

From an economic viewpoint, the new contract for hospital specialists is incomplete. Salaries remain the dominant payment mechanism, and explicit incentives for performance remain muted. Only the 'clinical excellence awards' can provide real incentives for activity, and these incentives may be limited in their operation unless well-defined criteria for their award are developed, and related clearly to overall NHS objectives. Attempts to supplement salaries with FFS to address variations and increase activity appear to have been marginalized in the contract reform, and therefore explicit and implicit incentives for performance remain deficient.

The new contract is based on remuneration of the hours specified in a 'job plan', where ten blocks of four hours are scheduled into 'programmed activities'. How well these hours and clinical activity in them are measured and managed will be determined by local hospitals. With only 40 hours per week superannuated, those already working longer hours may reduce their time input. Furthermore, activity within sessions will have to be monitored carefully as, in surgery in particular, activity rates appear to have been declining for some years. Even if consultant activity is stable after the contract reform, it remains likely that the activity rates of firms will decline due to reductions in the activity of more junior doctors, as they are affected by educational and working hours reforms.

The new GP contract

GP contracts are also very similar to those made at the inception of the NHS in 1948. In 1990, the Thatcher administration introduced GP fundholding and made marginal but important revisions to the contract, including some enhanced FFS payments and target payments. The current government has now proposed radical alterations to the contract (NHS Confederation and British Medical Association 2003). The new agreement is not contracted with individual practitioners but at practice level. Practices will be contracted to deliver varying levels of care: essential, additional and enhanced. The first two categories will normally be provided by all practices and will be funded with a global sum, paid to practices. Enhanced services will be subject to contract between the PCT and the practice. The basic contract will be for the period 08.00 until 18.30 hours during weekdays, and outside those hours there will be additional payments to practitioners. GPs who give up out-of-hours work will have their incomes reduced by £6,000 but may, if they wish, then contract with their PCT to do this work selectively, and perhaps with higher rewards.

Within the contract, practices will be rewarded for the achievement of 16 targets: 10 clinical, 5 managerial and 1 patient target. Practice-level rewards will be related to a system of points, the maximum of which will be 1050, with each point being worth a fixed amount of money.

How will activity be audited? The system appears to be highly dependent on trust. Investment in automated records and the creation, over time, of national record systems and performance review will help management of this expensive settlement. Patient satisfaction surveys may inform the local PCT about the existence and quality of service delivery, but it seems likely that regulatory bodies such as the Commission for Healthcare Audit and Inspection, the Audit Commission and the National Audit Office will require systematic and detailed data if they are to be convinced of value for money. The management challenge for PCTs is substantial.

How will quality be audited? The new contract will focus on primary care in isolation, rather than evaluation of the delivery of integrated, high-quality patient episodes of treatment. Linking primary care data with Hospital Episode Statistics, mortality data and health-related quality of life (HRQL) measures (e.g. as experimentally used by BUPA, see Vallance-Owen and Cubbin 2002) is required, but slow to be implemented.

The new contract will be delivered in part by GPs but also by the employment of even larger numbers of nurse practitioners in primary care. It is unclear how this increased demand for nurses will affect retention and recruitment in the hospital sector.

The new contract has been costed to fall within a defined expenditure. However, the 'knock-on' effects of the contract have not been quantified. Thus, as clinical targets are achieved, pharmaceutical and hospital costs may rise. For example, to treat and monitor high blood pressure it will be necessary to provide drugs (e.g. statins and beta blockers) and to test blood regularly in pathology. Many GPs will give up out-of-hours cover and lose £6,000 cash. However, such savings may be insufficient for PCTs to meet their statutory obligations for out-of-hours treatment by buying replacement specialist cover. The 'gap' could be met by skill dilution and the diversion of patients to hospital accident and emergency services.

The clinical standards set are systematic but not radically new. It is unclear, due to gross data deficits, how many practices meet these targets already and will only be rewarded for what they already do now. Some practices will move up to these standards. It is also unclear how practices will be developed beyond these standards in the future. There is an obvious risk that what is not incentivized will tend to be marginalized, regardless of its cost-effectiveness and value to patients. Pain control, services for drug users and incontinence services are potential examples.

The new GP contract contains a number of interesting innovations. The contract reform has focused almost exclusively on explicit incentives: essentially bonus payments and FFS. Implicit incentives, such as career concerns, remain relatively neglected. There is no real career structure for GPs in the NHS. The payment system created is complex, which, although it attempts to avoid any of the limitations of single system payment (e.g. salary, FFS or capitation alone), creates different risks. Two issues raised earlier are relevant. First, the more complex a pay system, the greater the scope for 'gaming' the system to maximize income. Over time, the complexity of the target payment system may mean that GPs can 'game' systems and increase their income (and hence NHS expenditure) by a 'points creep' upwards, similar to 'diagnostic-related-group (DRG) creep' which enabled US hospitals to 'harvest' payments product- ively. Second, it will be costly to keep the payment system up to date with technology changes and changes in patient demand. This could create inefficiency and inequity over time.

CONCLUSIONS

Incentives, explicit and implicit, are a means to an end – of using labour resources in order to achieve NHS efficiency and equity goals. Until now, both remuneration systems and the labour market in general have been poorly regulated due to inherent trust in the medical profession, reluctance of policymakers to engage in man- agement and monitoring, and their failure to articulate clearly the objectives of such regulation in terms of ensuring progression towards overall NHS goals. Now greater effort is being made to reform pay, the focus is largely to use capacity better (i.e. efficiency), with little attention being paid to equity goals. The design of pay- ment mechanisms to promote equity goals creates a new research agenda.

Substantial research challenges emerge from the current contract reforms. First, it is essential to evaluate the effect of the new con- tracts in relation to activity and outcome effects. A null hypothesis is that they are merely rents, and no substantive improvements in doctor performance are likely to be achieved. There is scope for rigorous quasi-experimental evaluation of the changes made. In add- ition, a substantial agenda of research is increasingly necessary in developing measures of performance based on patient outcomes, using this to develop improved methods of performance management.

There are some indications of weakening the obstacles to change in the regulation of the medical labour force, and of a gradual move- ment towards better management and measurement of activity and outcomes. For example, one Royal College is now recommending its members to validate their HES data (Williams and Mann 2002). While policies on safety and quality remain ill-defined, and face the risk of medical capture and bureaucratization, there is increasing recognition in research literature and some policy discussions of the need to use systematically available data to improve management of activity and outcomes. Methodological and managerial challenges in implementing this remain considerable.

Robinson (2001), in a review of physician payment and incentives in the USA, concludes that: 'In physician payment, as in most other aspects of life, matters are never as good as we might hope but never as bad as we might fear' (Robinson 2001: 174). This may be true in the UK: there may be scope for increases in overall performance, and for progress towards NHS efficiency and equity goals via the reform of medical contracts to change systems of financial incentives, and by improving information systems on which to base structures of management and regulation. However, careful evaluation of the impact of change is essential. Incentive structures, perhaps particularly in the medical market-place, are unlikely to have easily predictable effects due to the interweaving of explicit and implicit incentives, and to other factors influencing behaviour. Labour market responses to financial incentives, such as contract change, are always complex, and in medicine are further complicated by trust, duty and other influences. As summarized by Starr (1982: 3) 'the dream of reason did not take power into account'.

DISCUSSION
Anthony Scott

This chapter is a good overview of the role of incentives for doctors. The focus is on remuneration and explicit incentives, with less attention to labour market decisions and implicit incentives. The literature on personnel economics focuses more on career structures, promotion and internal labour markets, which have clear relevance in the health care labour market where salaried payment is common and where incentives for effort do exist if a dynamic perspective is taken. In focusing on consultants (fully qualified hospital specialists) and GPs, the chapter neglects the role of other members of the health care team, medical and non-medical. In particular, there may be career concerns and implicit incentives present for more junior doctors as well as incentives within teams, which could stimulate increased effort and activity.

A number of questions emerge, which may merit further research and exploration:

- the application of personnel economics to the health care labour market may be useful, reviewing career structures, incentives and internal labour markets;

- there may be potential for integrating better hospital activity data with workforce data, in order to assess the contribution of whole health care teams.
- there is still very little research on the interface between the public and private health sectors in the UK, which could be an important determinant of variation.
- the contract reform, for both hospital doctors and GPs, requires careful evaluation to assess whether behaviour changes and, if so, what the impact of this change is over time.

REFERENCES

Acheson, D. (1998) *Independent Inquiry into Inequalities in Health*. London: HMSO.

Andersen, T.F. and Mooney, G. (1990) *The Challenge of Medical Practice Variations*. London: Macmillan.

Appleby, J. (1996) Promoting efficiency in the NHS: problems with the labour productivity index, *British Medical Journal*, 313: 1319–21.

Arrow, K.J. (1963) Uncertainty and the welfare economics of medical care, *American Economic Review*, 53: 941–73.

Blomqvist, A. (1991) The doctor as double agent: information symmetry, health insurance and medical care, *Journal of Health Economics*, 10: 411–32.

Bloor, K., Maynard, A. and Freemantle, N. (2004) Variation in activity rates of consultant surgeons, and the influence of reward structures: descriptive analysis and a multi-level model, *Journal of Health Services Research and Policy* forthcoming.

Burgess, S. and Metcalfe, P. (1999) *Incentives in Organisations: A Selective Overview of the Literature with Application to the Public Sector*. CMPO Working Paper Series No. 00/16. Bristol: Leverhulme Centre for Market and Public Organisation.

Cabinet Office (1999) *Modernising Government*. London: The Stationery Office.

Commission for Health Improvement (2003) www.chi.gov.uk.

Department of Health (1999) *A First Class Service: Quality in the NHS*. London: HMSO.

Department of Health (2000) *The NHS Plan: A Plan for Investment, A Plan for Reform*. London: The Stationery Office.

Department of Health (2001a) *The NHS Plan: Proposal for a New Aproach to the Consultant Contract*. London: Department of Health.

Department of Health (2001b) *Rewarding Commitment and Excellence in the NHS – Consultation Document: Proposals for a New Consultant Reward Scheme*. Leeds: Department of Health.

Department of Health (2002) *A guide to NHS Foundation Trusts*. London: Department of Health.

Department of Health (2003) *Improving Rewards for NHS Consultants: A National Framework*, www.doh.gov.uk/consultantframework/ improvingrewardsguide.pdf, accessed September 2003.

Department of Health (2004) *NHS Reference Costs 2003 and National Tariff 2004*. London: Department of Health.

Department of Health & BMA Central Consultants and Specialists Committee (2002) *NHS Consultant Contract Framework 2002*, www.doh.gov.uk/ consultantframework/framework.pdf, accessed September 2003.

Dewatripont, M., Jewitt, I. and Tirole, J. (1999a) The economics of career concerns: part I, comparing information structures, *Review of Economic Studies*, 66: 183–98.

Dewatripont, M., Jewitt, I. and Tirole, J. (1999b) The economics of career concerns: part II, application to missions and accountability of government agencies, *Review of Economic Studies*, 66: 199–217.

Elliott, R.F. (1991) *Labor Economics: A Comparative Text*. Maidenhead: McGraw-Hill.

Evans, R.G. (1984) *Strained Mercy: The Economics of Canadian Health Care*. Toronto: Butterworth & Co.

Fisher, E.S., Wennberg, D.E., Stukel, T.A., Gottlieb, D.J., Lucas, F.L. and Pinder, E.L. (2003) The implications of regional variations in Medicare spending, part 2: health outcomes and satisfaction with care, *Ann Intern Med*, 138(4): 288–98.

Folland, S., Goodman, A.C. and Stano, M. (1993) *The Economics of Health and Health Care*. New York: Macmillan.

General Medical Council (2000) *Good Medical Practice*. London: General Medical Council.

Holmstrom, B. (1982a) Managerial incentive problems: a dynamic perspective. Essays in honour of Lars Wahlbeck, Helsinki, Finland. *Review of Economic Studies*, 66 (reprinted).

Holmstrom, B. (1982b) Moral hazard in teams, *Bell Journal of Economics*, 13: 324–40.

Kind, P., Dolan, P., Gudex, C. and Williams, A. (1998) Variations in population health status: results from a United Kingdom national questionnaire survey, *British Medical Journal*, 316: 736–41.

Maynard, A. and Bloor, K. (2003) Trust and performance management in the medical market place, *Journal of the Royal Society of Medicine*, 96: 532–9.

McGuire, T.G. (2000) Physician agency, in A.J. Culyer and J.P. Newhouse (eds) *Handbook of Health Economics*. Amsterdam: Elsevier.

McKeown, T. (1976) *The Role of Medicine: Dream, Mirage or Nemesis?* London: Nuffield Provincial Hospitals Trust.

McPherson, K., Wennberg, J.E., Hovind, O.B. and Clifford, P. (1982) Small area variations in the use of common surgical procedures: an international comparison of New England, England and Norway, *NEJM*, 307: 1310–14.

Newhouse, J.P. (1996) Reimbursing health plans and health providers: efficiency in production versus selection, *Journal of Economic Literature*, 34: 1236–63.

NHS Centre for Reviews and Dissemination (1996) *Hospital Volume and Health Care Outcomes, Costs and Patient Access (Effective Health Care, vol. 2, no. 8)*. York: University of York.

NHS Confederation and British Medical Association (2003) *New GMS Contract: Investing in General Practice*. London: NHS Confederation and BMA.

Office of Health Economics (2003) *Compendium of Health Statistics*. London: OHE.

O'Neill, O. (2002) A question of trust, in *The BBC Reith Lectures 2002*. Cambridge: Cambridge University Press.

Powell, J.E. (1966) *Medicine and Politics*. London: Pitman Medical.

Reinhardt, U.E. (1999) Reforming American health care: an interim report, *Journal of Rheumatology*, 26: 6–10.

Robinson, J.C. (1999) Blended payment methods in physician organizations under managed care, *Journal of the American Medical Association*, 282: 1258–63.

Robinson, J.C. (2001) Theory & practice in the design of physician payment incentives, *Milbank Quarterly*, 79: 149–77.

Smith, A. (1790) *A Theory of Moral Sentiments*. London: Oxford University Press.

Starr, P. (1982) *The Social Transformation of American Medicine: The Rise of Sovereign Profession and the Making of a Vast Industry*. New York: Basic Books.

Vallance-Owen, A. and Cubbin, S. (2002) Monitoring national clinical outcomes: a challenging programme, *British Journal of Health Care Management*, 8: 412–17.

Whynes, D.K. and Baines, D.L. (1998) Income-based incentives in UK general practice, *Health Policy*, 43: 15–31.

Williams, J.G. and Mann, R.Y. (2002) Hospital Episode Statistics: time for clinicians to get involved? *Clinical Medicine*, 2(1): 34–7.

Wilson, J.Q. (1989) *Bureaucracy: What Government Agencies Do and Why They Do It*. New York: Basic Books.

Yates, J. (1995) *Private Eye, Heart and Hip*. London: Churchill Livingstone.

8

FORMULA FUNDING OF HEALTH PURCHASERS: TOWARDS A FAIRER DISTRIBUTION?

Katharina Hauck, Rebecca Shaw and Peter C. Smith

INTRODUCTION

In most developed nations, the system of health care finance is used as an important instrument in seeking to secure a fair distribution of health care resources, and a system of 'capitation payments' is routinely used as the main basis for allocating health care expenditure to purchasing organizations (Rice and Smith 2001a). A capitation payment can be defined as the amount of health service funds associated with a citizen for a particular time period, and effectively puts a health care 'price' on the head of every citizen. Clearly the expected health care expenditure needs of citizens vary considerably, depending on personal characteristics such as age, morbidity and social circumstances. Considerable effort has therefore been expended on the process known as risk adjustment, which seeks to provide an unbiased estimate of the expected costs of a citizen relative to all other citizens.

One of the earliest developments in the use of capitation methods in the finance of health care was the work in England of the Resource Allocation Working Party in the 1970s (Resource Allocation Working Party 1976). This sought to allocate a fixed National Health Service (NHS) budget to geographical regions in accordance with an equity criterion of seeking to secure 'equal opportunity of access for those at equal risk'. The methods adopted by the Resource Allocation Working Party have been superseded by more empirically based approaches (Royston *et al.* 1992; Smith *et al.* 2001). However, the underlying equity objective has not changed, and is routinely used in most tax-based systems of health care throughout the developed world. Capitation methods are also commonly used where there is a competitive market of health care insurers, such as those found in many systems financed by social insurance (Van de Ven and Ellis 2000). Here the preoccupation is less with equity and more with minimizing the incentive for insurers to 'cream skim' only the healthiest patients within a particular risk group. However, the general policy priority remains unchanged – to seek to model the expected health care expenditure of a citizen with certain health, social and environmental characteristics.

However, for two reasons, the NHS has been reluctant merely to use unadjusted predictions of utilization as the basis for capitation payments. First, current utilization might, to some extent, reflect systematic variations in supply, implying that existing inequities might be perpetuated if no adjustment were made for such variations. Second, uncritical use of current utilization as the basis for setting capitation payments might introduce a perverse incentive for local agents to increase current utilization in order to attract higher capitation payments for their population in the future. These considerations have led to the development of a sophisticated econometric capitation methodology, principally on the basis of small area socioeconomic data (Carr-Hill *et al.* 1994; Sutton *et al.* 2002). Capitation methods in the UK have been the subject of intense scrutiny, and have influenced methods in a number of jurisdictions (Rice and Smith 2001a). They seek to identify the national average response, in terms of health care expenditure, to a set of local socioeconomic 'needs' indicators, after adjusting for supply factors.

Such approaches are intrinsically conservative, in the sense that they assume that (on average) the health system is currently meeting the desirable concept of need, whatever that concept might be (e.g. capacity to benefit, level of sickness, life expectancy and so on). The methods, therefore, fail to reflect 'legitimate' health care needs that are not currently met by the system. We do not intend to enter here into the debate about what is meant by need, although this clearly should be a germane focus of enquiry (Culyer 1995). For the purposes of this chapter, by using 'unmet need' we merely seek to indicate that certain groups of the population systematically fail to receive the health care that policymakers intend. The use of empirical utilization data as the basis of capitation payments is therefore inappropriate, as it perpetuates the inequity implied by the existence of unmet need, however need is defined (see Smith *et al.* 2001 for a discussion of these issues).

In the UK, the Labour government elected in May 1997 brought with it a policy of wishing to address persistent and growing inequalities in health. It set up an independent inquiry, chaired by Sir Donald Acheson, which recommended numerous policy options (Acheson 1998). It then produced a policy document, *Saving Lives: Our Healthier Nation* (Department of Health 1999) which put in place a public health agenda, with the objective of 'improving the health of everyone, especially the worst off' – that is, of improving health and reducing health inequalities. A review by Derek Wanless has reinforced the importance of public health issues for the long-term direction of the health system (Wanless 2004).

The commitment to reducing health inequalities in turn resulted in a reappraisal of the capitation criterion in use. The Advisory Committee on Resource Allocation, the body charged with developing capitation methodologies, was instructed by ministers to undertake a fundamental review of methods, incorporating a revised criterion for determining capitation payments to contribute to a reduction in avoidable health inequalities. This criterion represents a radical departure from that of seeking to offer equal opportunity of access, in effect seeking to secure a redistribution of health and implying that current practice was not securing outcomes in line with policy intentions. The criterion steers health policy quite determinedly away from the narrow concept of *health care* equity and towards the broader concept of *health* equity, with its implications for diverse policy areas such as income redistribution, housing, education, environment, transport and so on.

The purpose of this chapter is to put forward a simple economic model of health production, and to examine the implications of the new criterion for capitation methods. We start by developing a model of the traditional capitation criterion. We then go on to investigate various sources of inequality in health and discuss which of these can be addressed by a change in capitation methodology. The new capitation criterion is then introduced, and we discuss some of its political implications. Finally we offer some concluding comments.

A MODEL OF THE CURRENT CAPITATION CRITERION

In this section we explore, from a theoretical perspective, why inequalities in health might arise, and the implications for health care expenditure of seeking to reduce observed inequalities. The core of our exposition relies on an individual's health production function. This traces the efficient relationship between lifetime health care expenditure and health outcome, and is illustrated as the curve PP in Figure 8.1. For a given lifetime expenditure E on health care, and given current best clinical practice, the production function shows the maximum attainable health outcome (say life expectancy) Y of the individual. The maximum attainable life expectancy is Y*. The health production function is, of course, highly stylized, and requires careful examination before being used for analytic purposes.

First, we assume a single health care purchaser, which we call a 'National Health Service' (although the principles we set out are also valid for more devolved systems funded by capitation methods). In practice, other sources of health care (such as private sector providers) may be available. For the purposes of this chapter we think of these as being potential exogenous influences on the NHS production function shown in Figure 8.1. We also wish to sidestep the issue of which concept of 'health outcome' should be employed. The reader may wish to think of this as quality-adjusted life years. However, for expository purposes, we shall restrict discussion to a measure based on unadjusted life years. The choice of outcome measure does not materially affect the theoretical argument.

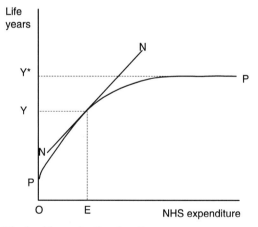

Figure 8.1　The health production function

We define health care expenditure to be lifetime expenditure by the NHS, discounted to birth. The capitation criterion under investigation is directed at health inequalities *avoidable by the NHS*, and we therefore concentrate on health outcomes that can be affected by that agency's actions. In specifying such a function we are, of course, presuming that extra health care activity can contribute to increased health, a claim that could be open to challenge. It is, moreover, important to acknowledge that there are many other exogenous factors that may influence the nature of the health production function and consequent inequalities. These include the individual's genetic characteristics, occupation, use of non-NHS health care, lifestyle and other external influences such as the environment, the economy and the actions of governmental and other, agencies. Changes in these factors might change the form of the NHS production function. For example, if an individual takes up a healthier lifestyle, this might give rise to an upward shift. We do not pursue these external influences further here, but it is worth noting that their inclusion in the model as a vector of circumstances is not, in principle, problematic.

Also, for ease of exposition, we assume a constant health care technology over the patient's lifetime. Of course, the rapid change in technologies that occurs in practice considerably complicates the practical problem for the health care system if it is to secure productive efficiency. This interesting issue is, however, not germane to this theoretical discussion. More generally, we restrict the analysis to the deterministic case, and do not introduce uncertainty arising from technologies, individual characteristics, external circumstances or NHS budget constraints. In practice, the effectiveness of health care is likely – to a greater or lesser extent – to fall some way short of the ideal indicated by the production function. *Random* inefficiencies of this sort do not materially affect the argument. *Systematically* larger inefficiencies suffered by particular groups relative to others are, however, discussed in some detail below.

The question now arises: given the shape of an individual's health production function, how much expenditure should the health care system devote to that individual? In systems that are not budget-constrained, we might, in principle, expect to observe expenditure up to the point where marginal benefit is zero. However, within a budget-constrained system of health care we must assume that some other criterion applies.

Many commentators argue that in these circumstances any decision rule for deciding how much to spend should be based on maximizing the health output of the system, given its budget constraint.

This principle gives rise to a simple decision rule: apply a uniform cut-off cost per life year saved, above which no treatment is offered. The cut-off can be represented by the slope of the line NN in Figure 8.1, which yields the optimal expenditure for the individual under scrutiny, given the global budget constraint. The same sloped line is applied to all individuals, whatever the shape of their health production functions. This model underlies almost all the literature on economic evaluation in health care and the use of health benefit measures such as quality-adjusted life years. There is probably a widespread consensus among health economists that it is – or at least ought to be – the principal efficiency criterion for allocating resources in health care (Culyer 1993). We term it the 'health maximization model'. It is important to note that – *if* we define need in terms of marginal capacity to benefit from health care – the health maximization model is consistent with the founding principle of the UK NHS (that those in equal need should have equal access to services) (Department of Health and Social Security 1976).

CAUSES OF INEQUALITIES IN HEALTH

Implicit in a capitation criterion of reducing health inequalities is the belief that currently health system resources are not being allocated in a socially desirable fashion. In particular, it suggests that, relative to their more healthy counterparts, the less healthy are receiving less health than is socially desirable. Three classes of circumstance might give rise to this state of affairs:

- systematic variations in health care quality (variations in technical efficiency);
- systematic variations in utilization of health care services (allocative inefficiency),
- systematic variations in health production functions (variations in people's efficiency in producing health).

We now consider these sources of inequality in turn, and we discuss which can be addressed by a change in capitation methodology.

Variations in health care quality

Suppose all individuals have the same production function and that the same cut-off criterion is applied to all individuals. That is, given the budget constraint, optimal expenditure E is being directed at all individuals. However, services for some classes of individual are technically inefficient in the sense that they offer poorer quality than those for healthier individuals – that is, outcomes lie below the production function frontier. This implies that treatments for two equally needy individuals differ due to variations in technical efficiency. This situation is represented in Figure 8.2 by the point L for the disadvantaged individual, giving rise to health outcome Y_L, as opposed to Y_H for the individual receiving better quality care.

Services to less healthy populations may be less technically efficient than other services for a number of reasons – expenditure may not be allocated optimally across an individual's lifetime, health care staff may be less motivated to secure good outcomes or may communicate poorly with less healthy individuals, recruitment of staff may be more difficult or capital configurations less appropriate in areas where the less healthy live, and so on. In this case, it is important to identify the true production possibilities, and to distinguish between improvements in outcome that can be secured by improved use of existing health care resources, and those that require additional resources. Addressing inequalities arising from technical inefficiency requires no change to capitation methods, because existing allocation of expenditure is optimal – it is the use of resources which is inefficient.

It is important to note, however, that this builds on the assumption that technical inefficiency is exogenous to the capitation system. It might be the case that the chosen capitation method provides an

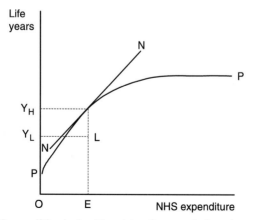

Figure 8.2 Inequalities in health arising from variations in technical efficiency for two individuals

incentive to behave inefficiently. For example, capitation payments positively weighted for the current sickness of the population could provide an incentive not to use resources efficiently for fear of improving the population's health status and thereby losing budget. For a discussion of behavioural responses on fixed budgets see Whynes *et al.* (1997), Shmueli and Glazer (1999) and Croxson *et al.* (2001).

For the purpose of this chapter we assume that inefficient behaviour is exogenous to the capitation system. Policy attention should therefore focus not on changing capitation methods, but on other instruments to secure better use of resources in services for disadvantaged populations. Countless types of quality initiative, such as the publication of comparative performance data, managerial incentive schemes and systems of audit and inspection, may help to secure progress towards this objective (Smith 2002).

Variations in utilization of health care services

Suppose that all individuals have the same production function and all are being treated technically efficiently (that is, on, rather than below, the production function). However, a stricter cut-off criterion is applied to some classes of individual than to others, implying the existence of allocative inefficiency. This may, for example, be due to market or informational failures on the demand or supply side of health care. Inequalities in utilization have the consequence that, although needs are identical, expenditure on health care is less for some groups than others. Figure 8.3 illustrates the principle for two

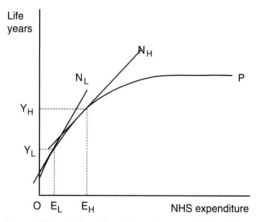

Figure 8.3   Inequalities in health arising from variations in access for two individuals

individuals, with the stricter treatment criterion applied to the disadvantaged individual L resulting in lower expenditure E_L and poorer outcome Y_L than for the other individual H. Under these circumstances, use of capitation payments E_L and E_H based on empirical data will perpetuate the implied inequity.

If a stricter cut-off criterion is currently being applied to some individuals than to others, a fundamental principle underlying many health care systems is being breached – that of equal access to health care for those in equal need. There is certainly evidence of considerable unmet need and of substantial inequalities in utilization in UK health care (Goddard and Smith 1998). Minority ethnic groups, disadvantaged socioeconomic groups, the elderly and persons living in remote areas experience inequalities, most notably in primary care, in prevention and health promotion, and in the treatment of coronary heart disease.

Inequalities in utilization unrelated to need imply that health maximization is not being secured, because the underserved have a greater capacity to benefit from expenditure than the relatively 'over-served'. A redirection of resources towards 'underserved' individuals is required, with an implication that capitation payments for disadvantaged populations should rise relative to the remainder of the population. This does not require definition of a new criterion for setting health care capitation payments. Rather, it requires the formulation of strategies aimed at eliminating allocative inefficiency in the provision of health care. The policy implication is, therefore, to design interventions that reduce utilization inequalities. The nature of these will, of course, be highly dependent on the reason for inequalities in access to services. In practice, very few studies have sought to address such policy issues (NHS Centre for Reviews and Dissemination 1995; Goddard and Smith 1998; Gordon *et al.* 1999).

For the purposes of capitation, attention should therefore focus on the magnitude of the associated unmet need, and on the expenditure consequences of rectifying the problem. In terms of Figure 8.3, the requirement is to quantify the shifts in expenditure $E_L E_H$ required to ensure that all citizens receive the same level of care. By definition, uncritical analysis of *existing* expenditure patterns will not yield useful information for this purpose. In principle, we should therefore seek out variations in the slope of the cut-off criterion applied to different social groups. In practice this is likely to be difficult. However, it may be that areas of the country exist where the unmet need has been eliminated, and that analysis of existing expenditure patterns within those areas may yield an acceptable basis for setting national capitation payments. Sutton and Lock (2000) show how this could be done in a Scottish context although the rather arbitrary method of selecting 'exemplar' areas adopted in that study indicates the type of practical problems likely to be encountered. Of course, even if capitation payments can be corrected to account for unmet need, there remains a performance management problem of ensuring that the increased funds associated with unmet need are indeed directed towards the currently underserved population.

Variations in health production functions

Suppose that all individuals are being treated with technical and allocative efficiency, in accordance with the health maximization model. However, individuals have different health production functions, so that their health outcomes vary. This situation is illustrated in Figure 8.4, which compares two individuals with different health profiles, in the sense that – at the same level of health expenditure – individual L is unambiguously less healthy than individual H. This is due to determinants of health that are beyond the immediate influence of the health services, such as the social and economic environment, genetic endowments or lifestyle choices of the individuals concerned. The cut-off criterion is indicated by the slope of the straight lines, and gives rise to health outcomes Y_H and Y_L. The implied capitation payments are E_H and E_L. Application of an equal

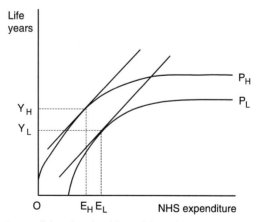

Figure 8.4 Inequalities in health arising from different production functions for two individuals

cut-off criterion implies smaller health inequalities in comparison to an equal allocation of expenditure to H and L.

If all patients are being treated in accordance with the health maximization principle, but the outcome is nevertheless unacceptable, then a reallocation of resources according to some equity criterion is required, under which resources are redirected towards less healthy individuals. Avoidable inequalities of this sort arise, even though quality of and access to health care are equal for identical citizens, because of differences between individuals that are outside the control of the health services. Policy attention to such inequalities reflects a concern with principles of *vertical* equity between individuals, rather than the traditional concern with *horizontal* equity embedded in most capitation methodology (Rice and Smith 2001b). In principle, society should address vertical equity issues by considering an optimal reallocation of all resources, both private and public. However, our focus is purely on the health care sector, and in this context the unacceptable health inequalities imply that a fundamental revision of capitation methods may, therefore, be required.

A MODEL OF THE NEW CAPITATION CRITERION

Policy to correct for variations in people's efficiency in producing health implies an interest in increasing the level of health care for the less healthy relative to that received by the healthy in order to compensate for such disadvantage. As in the case of allocative inefficiency, this implies a shift of health care resources in the form of capitation payments towards the less healthy. In contrast, however, the objective here is to rectify a perceived injustice in individual endowments, and not inefficiencies within the health care system. In the extreme case of wishing to *eliminate* avoidable health inequalities, a situation as in Figure 8.5 might arise. Expenditure on individual L is increased in order to secure the same life span as currently enjoyed by individual H. This results in increased capitation payment E_L^*. Note that the marginal cost per life year saved becomes higher for individual L (the associated line $N_L N_L$ becomes shallower than the original NN). This might imply that the unhealthy individual receives treatments which the healthy individual does not receive, or that the unhealthy individual receives more expensive treatments, or treatments of a higher quality.

The situation set out in Figure 8.5 would result in an unambiguous rise in the health care budget requirement. If this were considered

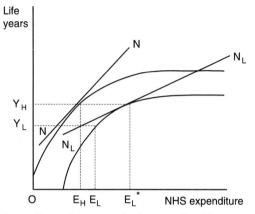

Figure 8.5   Expenditure change required to equalize life expectancy

unrealistic, the solution would be simultaneously to reduce expenditure on individual H while increasing expenditure on individual L. That is, health inequalities would be reduced partially by *worsening* the outcome for healthier individuals. In Figure 8.5, a revenue-neutral solution would then result in a common life expectancy somewhere between Y_H and Y_L (although whether this is politically feasible is another matter!).

The strategy of *eliminating* avoidable mortality is, of course, extreme. In practice, both limited technological capacity and strength of public preferences might give rise to a policy reluctance to seek to eliminate variations entirely. A more realistic criterion is, therefore, to *reduce* avoidable inequality. Figure 8.6 shows a situation where some unhealthy individuals are unable to achieve the same life span as individual H, in which case the health services would – under the criterion of 'eliminating avoidable inequality' – spend up to the point where the marginal benefit of health care expenditure and the slope of the cut-off is zero. The remaining inequalities – symbolized by the distance between Y_H and Y_L – could only be eliminated by reducing the health status of individual H. If this is politically undesirable, the remaining inequalities are deemed politically 'unavoidable'.

It is likely that a broader view of social policy would indicate that interventions in other public policy areas – such as housing, public transport or income redistribution – are effective in eliminating health inequalities. Successful policies in other areas would result in an upward shift of the health production function in Figure 8.6. This

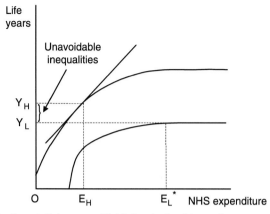

Figure 8.6   Inequalities unavoidable by the health services

argument can be extended to the case where it is possible, but inefficient, to reduce inequalities with health care interventions. In a situation where inequalities in health could be further reduced only with
very high health care expenditure, public expenditure in other policy
areas might lead to exogenous improvements in health production.
This combination of strategies may require less public expenditure
than a strategy based solely on health care policy. In order to make
this assessment, the marginal effectiveness in reducing inequalities in
health of alternative public policies (and possibly even portfolios of
policies) should be compared. In principle, a socially optimal health
inequalities policy would allocate resources across policy areas so
that the marginal benefit of public expenditure (in terms of reducing
health inequalities) would be equal in each policy area.

Another reason why society might not want to adopt the complete elimination of inequalities as an objective is that it entails a
sacrifice in overall population health. For any set budget, any
attempt to reduce health inequalities results in less total health gain
than in the health maximization model outlined above. The more
equal life expectancy under the new capitation criterion is less than
the average of Y_H and Y_L. The policymaker's problem now becomes
one of balancing total health gain (an efficiency objective) against
reductions in inequalities (an equity objective) (Wagstaff 1991;
Williams 1997). The problem is illustrated in Figure 8.7, which traces
the health production possibilities arising from the health production functions for two individuals with different levels of health. (The
appendix – p. 215 – shows how Figure 8.7 can be derived from the

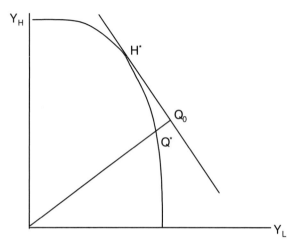

Figure 8.7   The health production possibility frontier

individual production functions.) Figure 8.7 indicates – for a fixed budget constraint – the possible mixes of maximum health outcomes Y_L and Y_H that the NHS could in principle secure for the two individuals. The point H* indicates the maximum aggregate health attainable for the two individuals subject to the given budget constraint. The point Q* is the point where the two would secure equal health, and the distance $Q*Q_0$ indicates the aggregate loss in health brought about by pursuit of such pure equality. In practice, it seems likely that there exists a social welfare function (SWF) which results in a policy intermediate between the points Q* and H*, reflecting the politically preferred balance between efficiency and equity objectives.

Any system for setting capitation payments requires a clear normative definition of the concept of equity in health that policymakers have in mind. Any deviation from the health maximization criterion may imply that individuals with the same capacity to benefit from health care receive different amounts of health care resources. Unequal treatments require political justification, and this is the role of the equity concept. There is a substantial, if not always enlightening, theoretical economics literature on equity concepts in health and health care (Williams and Cookson 2000), but there has been little empirical examination of what meanings or precise specifications stakeholders attach to the concept (Pereira 1989). Therefore, it will be difficult to find agreement on a particular equity concept. Moreover, once identified, the theoretical equity concept needs to be translated into an unambiguous resource allocation pattern. This is, without doubt, an acute political problem (Culyer and Wagstaff 1993).

Finally, it is worth noting that the new capitation method implies better medical treatment of unhealthy groups of the population. This gives rise to major practical difficulties in defining criteria for membership of the targeted group, and ensuring that health care is delivered in accordance with policy intentions. Furthermore, it might result in incentives for individuals to acquire membership of those groups that are given privileged access. The variety of practical difficulties that emerge when seeking to make operational principles of vertical equity – as distinct from horizontal equity – are considered elsewhere (Mooney 1996).

CONCLUSIONS

This chapter has sought to link the economic literature on health inequalities with the policy issue of capitation payments when there is interest in using the funding system to address public health concerns. It has demonstrated that there are three broad categories of causes of health inequality relevant to the health sector: variations in efficiency, variations in access to care and variations in personal health production. This last poses the most fundamental challenge to capitation policy, as addressing it implies a desire to move away from a policy of equality of access (horizontal equity) towards one of targeting health care at particular classes of individual (vertical equity). There is clearly a major challenge in seeking out the evidence on which the change to the capitation methods would be based. Two broad classes of information required relate to the effectiveness of interventions in reducing health inequalities, and public preferences regarding the importance of reducing health inequalities. Both sorts of evidence are in short supply (Lindholm *et al.* 1998; Andersson and Lyttkens 1999).

Furthermore, there is no guarantee that mere alteration of capitation payments will ensure that additional resources reach deprived populations. By definition, the vertical equity criterion requires that the health sector alters the way in which it delivers health care to those with poor health expectancy. Yet, in general, directing extra 'health inequality' resources at needy areas will not necessarily lead to reduction in health inequalities. Rather, it may merely lead to the perpetuation of existing patterns of utilization in an area, albeit at a higher level than before. Important performance management and auditing issues are therefore raised if the policy reflected in the revised capitation payments is to be translated into desired action by health care professionals. We have very little evidence on 'what works' in this respect (Macintyre 2003), and there is a clear need for better evaluation of public health initiatives.

The discussion has emphasized the role of health services in addressing public health, and has made only general reference to the broader influences of social policy on inequalities. This emphasis reflects the current administrative reality – that health ministries perceive their principal role to be one of delivering health care. Yet there is no reason in principle why health ministries should not be responsible for addressing the health inequality implications of *all* areas of public policy. Under this arrangement they would be responsible for auditing the impact on health inequalities of major public sector initiatives, and for levying 'taxes' (or providing subsidies) to encourage policies that contribute to health inequality policy. Nurturing this role would be one approach towards the optimal distribution of all public resources.

It is also important to note that an emphasis on health inequalities offers a profound challenge to the evaluation of health care technology. In principle, it implies that technologies should be evaluated differently according to the health status of the individual – that is, the need to target certain unhealthy groups may mean that certain treatments are recommended for those groups that are not considered cost-effective for healthier groups. This consideration complicates the task of designing and evaluating trials enormously, and implies a move towards Williams' (1999) notion of equity-adjusted quality-adjusted life years as the basis for economic evaluation. The principle also offers considerable challenges in framing intelligible clinical guidelines for practitioners. Yet the logic of incorporating a health inequality criterion into resource allocation leads inevitably to its incorporation into economic evaluation of technologies, with all the attendant complications.

Thus, seeking to amend capitation payments to address public health concerns raises many challenging issues relating to the distribution of resources in health care and the broader public services. However, we believe that the economic models presented here offer a systematic and coherent framework for addressing these challenges.

ACKNOWLEDGEMENT

An earlier version of this chapter appeared in *Health Economics*, 11(8): 667–77.

APPENDIX: DERIVATION OF THE HEALTH PRODUCTION POSSIBILITY FRONTIER

This appendix indicates how the (two person) production possibility frontier can be derived from the individual health production functions. The production frontiers for person H and person L are replicated (in a transposed state) in the top left and bottom right corners of the diagram respectively. The fixed expenditure budget constraint $E_H + E_L$ is represented by the straight line in the bottom left quadrant. All expenditure choices must conform to this constraint. They are then reflected, via the production functions, into the top right quadrant, which therefore yields the production possibility frontier, which is reproduced as Figure 8.7 in the main text.

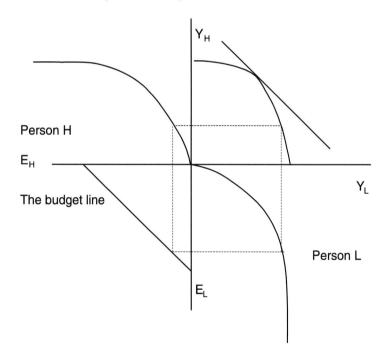

DISCUSSION
Matt Sutton

Chapter 8 provides an insightful framework for the discussion of how capitation funding formulae can address health inequalities. As noted in several places the evidence base for many of the major issues is sparse. In practice, attempts to make funding formulae 'fairer' have concentrated on addressing (differentially) unmet need – the second of the scenarios presented in the chapter.

My discussion reviews these practical developments. First, clarification is given of the term 'unmet need'. Second, the ways in which formulae cope with unmet need are described. The final section reviews recent attempts to correct for unmet need.

WHAT IS UNMET NEED?

Fundamental problems with the new capitation objective in the UK are the lack of clarity about how health care resources are intended to reduce inequalities in health and the dearth of evidence upon which to base these decisions. While there is a large evaluation industry for the effect of interventions on health, there is little evidence on how health care inputs affect health at the aggregate level. The few available studies adopt either inventory approaches in specific disease areas (Capewell *et al.* 1999) or weakly powered and probably confounded correlational analysis of observational data at the aggregate level (Guilford 2002).

More fundamentally, there are two ways to *interpret* the new objective: (i) the NHS budget should be allocated to reduce inequalities in health and health care organizations need to invest in health care or other interventions so as to reduce health inequalities most efficiently, or (ii) the budget should be allocated according to need, regardless of whether these needs *tend* to be met. In the latter case, inequities in health care are believed to exacerbate inequalities in health and the budget should be allocated so that inequities in health care can be reduced. The health care sector is required only to 'put its own house in order' and ensure that the distribution of health care resources no longer contributes deleteriously to inequalities in health, rather than compensate for the effects of other factors.

In practice, the UK formula has moved from attempts at the former to the latter interpretation and this history is reviewed below. I do not review evidence of inequities in health care, which is a voluminous, but rather inconsistent, literature that has been reviewed elsewhere (Propper 1998; Goddard and Smith 2001; Dixon *et al.* 2003). This discussion is confined mainly to experience in the UK – the international practice of formula funding has been reviewed elsewhere (Rice and Smith 2001a).

HOW DO STANDARD FORMULAE COPE WITH UNMET NEED?

The first empirically based formula in England took account of additional need through a single indicator – the Standardized Mortality Ratio 0–64 years. This indicator was plausible and pragmatically chosen, and was assumed to have a proportional relationship with need. The weighting was subsequently reviewed and, as a more sophisticated understanding of the multi-dimensional nature of populations and their health care needs developed, the formula was extended to reflect multiple variables. This required a method for selecting and weighting variables (sometimes called the 'calibration' of the model) which gave rise to utilization-based formulae, in which small-area variations in health care use were estimated as a function of need and supply indicators (Carr-Hill *et al.* 1994).

This represented a substantial step forward, but used the current relationship between population characteristics and health care consumption to calibrate the formula. While the first formula was somewhat arbitrary and judgement-based, it was unaffected by unmet need since it paid no attention to health care consumption. The formulae presented by Carr-Hill *et al.*, on the other hand, implicitly built any systematic unmet need into future funding. If the needs of particular groups were unmet or 'under-met' then the related population characteristic had a coefficient that was either negative, zero or underestimated. Although in the Carr-Hill formulae there was the potential for unmet need caused by under-supply to be identified, the final estimation approach precluded this (Gravelle *et al.* 2003).

These arguments are not just theoretical. In the acute services formula, the proportion in black ethnic groups was found to be negative. Conditional on other variables, this effect was interpreted as evidence of unmet need. Accordingly, this variable was dropped and the model was re-run so that areas with higher proportions of black people did not receive less resources directly. But dropping counter-intuitive variables and re-running the model converts unmet need into an omitted variables problem, and variables with which it is positively correlated will be assigned reduced coefficients. Therefore, the estimated formula is conservative, because it continues to reflect currently unmet need – albeit indirectly. This is not just a problem of the small-area approach but also of the matrix approach based on individual-level data (Smith *et al.* 2001). For example, Diderichsen's treatment of the observed deficit for immigrants in Stockholm County also left some element of unmet need implicit in the chosen formula (Diderichsen *et al.* 1997).

ADJUSTMENTS FOR UNMET NEED

Initial attempts to cope with the new capitation objective in the UK followed the same pattern as the original approaches to resource allocation. An indicator of poor population health (premature years of life lost) was pragmatically selected and the weighting (this time in terms of the number of areas to benefit and the size of the budget affected) arbitrarily agreed.

The recent review of the formula was tasked with devising an empirical adjustment for unmet need (Sutton *et al.* 2002). In this review, unexpected negative coefficients were interpreted as unmet need (if supported by individual-level analysis and the effect judged not to be generated by multi-collinearity), and allocations were based on the other variables evaluated in a model allowing for unmet need (Schokkaert and Van de Voorde 2000). For example, in the acute sector model, ethnicity and unemployment were found to have negative coefficients and the effect of adjusting for unmet need resulted in a needs index that was 28 per cent steeper than the one in which these variables were dropped and the model re-run (Gravelle *et al.* 2003).

A review of resource allocation in Wales (National Assembly for Wales Health and Social Services Committee 2001) pursued a method that was also sold as avoiding problems of unmet need. Prevalence estimates were obtained for each area and resources were allocated on the basis of each area's share of national prevalence. However, the simplicity of the method, which was partly determined by a lack of quality data on health care use, is beguiling. It suffers from similar limitations to the first English formula – the conditions for which prevalence estimates were obtained was a pragmatic selection and resources were allocated in proportion to the prevalence estimates. The strong assumptions of this method were illustrated and debated in an exchange of papers in the *Journal of Health Economics* in 1991 in the context of measuring equity in health care (Le Grand 1991; Wagstaff *et al.* 1991). Need is assumed to be determined only by the absence of a particular health condition – individuals without the condition are assumed to have no need and all people with the condition are assumed to have the same level of need for health care resources. It is not difficult to show that the choice of health measure (even for an apparently specific disease area) can have a substantial effect on allocations to each area with the prevalence of more minor conditions resulting in narrower differences (McConnachie and Sutton 2004). For these reasons, proposals for this to be adopted in England (Asthana *et al.* 2004) should be resisted.

The advantage of deriving adjustments for unmet need within the utilization model framework is that *evidence* of unmet need is simultaneously produced. The approach is to *test* for inequity in health care and, *if* evidence of its existence is found, adjustments can be made to ensure it is not reflected in the allocations. This approach is becoming increasingly popular – in Scotland, for example, an adjustment to the formula to reflect inequities in health care was published earlier in 2004 (McConnachie and Sutton 2004). Scotland's formula has only one (composite) needs indicator – the Arbuthnott Index. The unmet need adjustment was derived in two stages: (i) estimated prevalence rates for small areas were obtained by analysing the relationships between prevalence rates in a health survey and the Arbuthnott Index; and (ii) variations in health care utilization between small areas were modelled as a function of these estimated prevalence rates, with tests for higher or lower levels of met need in the highest and lowest need areas.

The organizations that would gain under such an adjustment have been required to bid for funds and the released monies will be subject to evaluation. However, why these particular funds have been singled out is unclear. Organizations are not held accountable for, or even monitored on, how they distribute resources between areas or population groups, despite evidence of considerable variation in the distribution of resources across national indicators of need (Sutton and Lock 2000; Sutton *et al.*

2002). The selection of certain organizations as examples of good practice has been considered in Scotland and England for making unmet need adjustments, but never applied. Variations in the extent to which health care organizations distribute their funding in line with need thwart the equity objectives of the national formula. Understanding how these variations arise is probably the next major challenge in this area.

REFERENCES

Acheson, D. (1998) *Independent Inquiry into Inequalities in Health*. London: HMSO.

Andersson, F. and Lyttkens, C.H. (1999) Preferences for equity in health behind a veil of ignorance, *Health Economics*, 8: 369–78.

Asthana, S., Gibson, A., Moon, G., Dicker, J. and Brigham, P. (2004) The pursuit of equity in NHS resource allocation: should morbidity replace utilisation as the basis for setting health care capitations? *Social Science and Medicine*, 58: 539–551.

Capewell, S., Morrison, C.E. and McMurray, J.J. (1999) Contribution of modern cardiovascular treatment and risk factor changes to the decline in coronary heart disease mortality in Scotland between 1975 and 1994, *Heart*, 81: 380–6.

Carr-Hill, R.A., Sheldon, T.A., Smith, P., Martin, S., Peacock, S. and Hardman, G. (1994) Allocating resources to health authorities: development of methods for small area analysis of use of inpatient services, *British Medical Journal*, 309: 1046–9.

Croxson, B., Propper, C. and Perkins, A. (2001) Do doctors respond to financial incentives? UK family doctors and the GP fundholding scheme, *Journal of Public Economics*, 79(2): 375–98.

Culyer, A.J. (1993) Health, health expenditures and equity, in F. Rutten (ed.) *Equity in the Finance and Delivery of Health Care: An International Perspective*. Oxford: Oxford University Press.

Culyer, A.J. (1995) Need – the idea won't do – but we still need it, *Social Science and Medicine*, 40(6): 727–30.

Culyer, A.J. and Wagstaff, A. (1993) Equity and equality in health and health care, *Journal of Health Economics*, 12: 431–7.

Department of Health (1999) *Saving Lives: Our Healthier Nation*. London: The Stationery Office.

Department of Health and Social Security (1976) *Sharing Resources for Health in England: Report of the Resource Allocation Working Party*. London: HMSO.

Diderichsen, F., Varde, E. and Whitehead, M. (1997) Resource allocation to health authorities: the quest for an equitable formula in Britain and Sweden, *British Medical Journal*, 315: 875–8.

Dixon, A., Le Grand, J., Henderson, J., Murray, R. and Poteliakhoff, E. (2003) *Is the NHS Equitable? A Review of the Evidence.* LSE Health Discussion Paper 11. London: London School of Economics.

Goddard, M. and Smith, P. (1998) *Equity of Access to Health Care.* York: Centre for Health Economics, University of York.

Goddard, M. and Smith, P. (2001) Equity of access to health care services: theory and evidence from the UK, *Social Science and Medicine*, 53(9): 1149–62.

Gordon, D., Shaw, M., Dorling, D. and Davey-Smith, G. (1999) *Inequalities in Health: The Evidence Presented to the Independent Inquiry into Inequalities in Health, Chaired by Sir Donald Acheson.* Bristol: The Policy Press.

Gravelle, H., Sutton, M., Morris, S., Windmeijer, F., Leyland, A., Dibben, C. and Muirhead, M. (2003) Modelling supply and demand influences on the use of health care: implications for deriving a needs-based capitation formula, *Health Economics*, 12(12): 985–1004.

Guilford, C. (2002) Availability of primary care doctors and population health in England: is there an association? *Journal of Public Health Medicine*, 24: 252–4.

Le Grand, J. (1991) The distribution of health care revisited: a commentary on Wagstaff, van Doorslaer and Paci, and O'Donnell and Propper, *Journal of Health Economics*, 10: 239–45.

Lindholm, L., Rosen, M. and Emmelin, M. (1998) How many lives is equity worth? A proposal for equity adjusted years of life saved, *Journal of Epidemiological Community Health*, 52: 808–11.

Macintyre, S. (2003) Evidence-based policy making, *British Medical Journal*, 326: 5–6.

McConnachie, A. and Sutton, M. (2004) *Derivation of an Adjustment to the Arbuthnott Formula for Socioeconomic Inequities in Health Care.* Edinburgh: Scottish Executive.

Mooney, G. (1996) And now for vertical equity? Some concerns arising from aboriginal health in Australia, *Health Economics*, 5: 99–103.

National Assembly for Wales Health and Social Services Committee (2001) *Targeting Poor Health: Professor Townsend's Report of the Welsh Assembly's National Steering Group on the Allocation of NHS Resources.* Cardiff: National Assembly for Wales.

NHS Centre for Reviews and Dissemination (1995) *Review of Research on the Effectiveness of Health Service Interventions to Reduce Variations in Health.* York: Centre for Reviews and Dissemination.

Pereira, J. (1989) *What Does Equity in Health Mean?* Discussion Paper 61. York: University of York Centre for Health Economics.

Propper, C. (1998) *Who Pays for and Who Gets Health Care? Equity in the Finance and Delivery of Health Care in the United Kingdom.* Nuffield Occasional papers, Health Economics Series No. 5. London: The Nuffield Trust.

Resource Allocation Working Party (1976) *Sharing Resources for Health in England.* London: HMSO.

Rice, N. and Smith, P. (2001a) Capitation and risk adjustment in health care financing: an international progress report, *The Milbank Quarterly*, 79(1): 81–113.

Rice, N. and Smith, P.C. (2001b) Ethics and geographical equity in health care, *Journal of Medical Ethics*, 27(4): 256–61.

Royston, G.H.D., Hurst, J.W., Lister, E.G. and Stewart, P.A. (1992) Modelling the use of health services by populations of small areas to inform the allocation of central resources to larger regions, *Socio-Economic Planning Sciences*, 26(3): 169–80.

Schokkaert, E. and Van de Voorde, C. (2000) *Risk Selection and the Specification of the Conventional Risk Adjustment Formula*. Centre for Economic Studies Discussion Paper DPS 00.11. (www.econ.kuleuven.ac.be/ew/admin/Publications/DPS00/DPS0011.pdf). Leuven: KULeuven.

Shmueli, A. and Glazer, J. (1999) Addressing the inequity of capitation by variable soft contracts, *Health Economics*, 8(4): 335–43.

Smith, P. (2002) Performance management in British health care: will it deliver? *Health Affairs*, 21(3): forthcoming.

Smith, P., Rice, N. and Carr-Hill, R. (2001) Capitation funding in the public sector, *Journal of the Royal Statistical Society, Series A*, 164(2): 217–57.

Sutton, M. and Lock, P. (2000) Regional differences in health care delivery: implications for a national resource allocation formula, *Health Economics*, 9(6): 547–59.

Sutton, M., Gravelle, H., Morris, S., Leyland, A., Windmeijer, F., Dibben, C. and Muirhead, M. (2002) *Allocation of Resources to English Areas: Individual and Small Area Determinants of Morbidity and Use of Healthcare Resources*. Edinburgh: ISD Consultancy Services.

Van de Ven, W.P.M.M. and Ellis, R. (2000) Risk adjustment in competitive health plan markets, in A.J. Culyer (ed.) *Handbook of health economics*. Amsterdam: Elsevier.

Wagstaff, A. (1991) QALYs and the equity-efficiency trade-off. *Journal of Health Economics*, 10: 21–41.

Wagstaff, A., van Doorslaer, E. and Paci, P. (1991) Horizontal equity in the delivery of health care, *Journal of Health Economics*, 10: 251–6.

Wanless, D. (2004) *Securing our Future Health: Taking a Long Term View*. London: HM Treasury.

Whynes, D., Heron, T. and Avery, A. (1997) Prescribing cost savings by GP fundholders: long term or short term? *Health Economics*, 8: 335–43.

Williams, A. (1997) Beyond effectiveness and efficiency . . . lies equality! in I. Chalmers (ed.) *Non-random Reflections on Health Services Research*. London: BMJ Publishing Group.

Williams, A. (1999) Intergenerational equity: an exploration of the 'fair innings' argument, *Health Economics*, 8: 1–8.

Williams, A. and Cookson, R. (2000) Equity in health, in J. Newhouse (ed.) *Handbook of Health Economics*. Amsterdam: Elsevier.

9

DECENTRALIZATION IN HEALTH CARE: LESSONS FROM PUBLIC ECONOMICS

Rosella Levaggi and Peter C. Smith

INTRODUCTION

The most appropriate decentralization of policymaking powers is an important unresolved policy question for most health systems. At one extreme lies the UK National Health Service (NHS), in which the central authority sets most policies, and lower levels have little room for manoeuvre regarding the nature or financing of services. At the other extreme lies the USA, with a pluralistic web of purchasers and providers, and little central policy of any effectiveness.

The difficulty of commanding a health system from the centre has led many systems to explore the potential for decentralizing powers to lower levels of government. Traditional NHS-type systems such as Italy and Spain have devolved health system policymaking and finance to regions covering populations of about 3 million people (Reverte-Cejudo and Sanchez-Bayle 1999). In the UK, the systems of Wales, Scotland and Northern Ireland are beginning to diverge following the introduction of devolution (Pollock 1999), and policymakers are – at least in their rhetoric – beginning to promote greater decentralization of NHS powers within England (Department of Health 2003). In contrast, countries such as Norway and Portugal are currently moving towards more centralization of powers (World Health Organization 2003). Decentralization has also been an important unresolved element of health system design in many developing countries (Mills 1994; World Bank 2003).

Many health systems have traditionally delegated substantial powers. In Scandinavian countries a large degree of responsibility for the health system is vested in local government (Koivusalo 1999). Federal countries, such as Canada and Australia, have made provinces or states the principal locus of health policymaking (Armstrong and Armstrong 1999). Yet it is worth noting that – even in these well-established, decentralized systems – the national government often retains considerable powers of oversight and regulation, and there remain important tensions about where the balance of responsibility for the health system should lie (Lazar *et al.* 2002).

Some proponents appear to view decentralization as an unambiguously virtuous ambition. Yet the ultimate logic of decentralization is that responsibility for health and health care should be devolved to the household. The manifestly dysfunctional nature of health systems that promote this principle (most notably the USA) should therefore alert us to the danger of a blind pursuit of decentralization. While a degree of decentralization down to some level of collective authority may indeed yield substantial gains for the health system, pursued excessively there can be no doubt that decentralization in health care leads to serious difficulties.

Economists have developed a substantial literature on the topic of decentralized public services, usually referred to under the banner of 'fiscal federalism' (Oates 1999). This literature focuses on the optimal administrative level at which to vest powers of finance and purchasing of public services, and examines the consequences of alternative distributions of responsibilities. It therefore seems very germane to recent debates on decentralization in health care, though to date there have been few English language analyses of the implications of the fiscal federalism literature for health system design (see Petretto 2000 for an exception).

This chapter seeks to correct this. We first offer some brief comments on what is meant by decentralization in health care. The next section introduces the economic view of decentralization, and sets out the major economic arguments adduced in the decentralization debate. We then focus on three key issues: the diversity of health systems that may arise under decentralization; the role of information in decentralization; and the coordination needs of decentralized services. The main contribution of economic models is to offer a framework for thinking about decentralization, rather than any firm policy prescriptions. The chapter concludes with a discussion of what we feel are the key judgements needed to develop effective policy towards decentralization.

The discussion is quite broad, and is concerned mainly with the purchasing of health services. In practice, local providers, most especially hospitals, are often in the driving seat of local health services, and the purchasing function is weak. However, we believe this reality reflects a failure of local governance, and that it is the purchasing function with which local communities should be preeminently concerned. We leave open the question of who should provide the services. Moreover, health care is hugely diverse in both the tasks it undertakes and the technologies it deploys. It is therefore highly likely that an organizational structure that is good for some health system tasks may be less satisfactory for others.

Throughout we refer loosely to 'local government'. This is merely shorthand for a sub-national institution that enjoys a certain amount of autonomy in setting priorities and (possibly) raising revenue, and is not intended to refer necessarily to existing local government arrangements (such as local authorities in the UK). The local government under discussion could range in size from Australian states to Finnish municipalities. Also, how the governors of the local institution are appointed is left open. However, our usual assumption is that they are subject to periodic popular local elections, in contrast (say) to being appointed by a national minister.

WHAT IS DECENTRALIZATION IN HEALTH CARE?

Decentralization in health care is difficult to define. However, in broad terms it entails the transfer of powers from a central authority (typically the national government) to more local institutions. Given the immense complexity of health and health care and the associated governance arrangements, it is possible to envisage infinite variety in the nature and strength of any decentralization, embracing considerations as diverse as political autonomy, service provision, representation, finance and legal frameworks. Saltman *et al.* (2003) cite four types of decentralization: delegation, de-concentration, devolution and privatization. Delegation transfers responsibility to a lower organizational level, de-concentration to a lower administrative level and devolution to a lower political level, while privatization takes place when tasks are transferred from public to private ownership.

In this chapter we do not dwell on these subtly different notions of decentralization, which may have radically different implications for system behaviour. A full treatment of decentralization would require commentaries from a number of perspectives, including political, psychological, sociological and clinical. Instead we comment from an economic perspective on just two issues that are common to all types of decentralization: transfer of finance powers and transfer of policy powers.

The extent to which local institutions are given autonomy over how they can raise and use finance is a central design decision in any decentralization policy. At one extreme, localities may be assigned a fixed budget by the national government and allowed no fiscal autonomy at all. Indeed, the national government may subdivide the budget so that expenditure on certain specific activities is 'ring-fenced'. Local choice then becomes one of deciding a preferred pattern of services within the fixed budget. At the other extreme, local governments may be free to use any local tax base they choose (e.g. the voters of Seattle were recently asked to consider a ten-cent 'coffee tax') and to set any level of tax rates. In health care, an important autonomous source of finance may be charges for service users, which in this context can be considered a tax on the sick.

Similarly, local governments may at one extreme have absolute autonomy over the policies they adopt, or they may be subject to strong central regulations on (say) minimum standards, and at the extreme, become mere agents for the national government. In short, it is important to distinguish between the nominal degree of decentralization and the real extent of local autonomy. In health care, national governments almost invariably insist on certain minimum standards, often in the form of a 'basic package'. Localities may then be free, at the margin, to enhance the package or alter user charges. Any variations from national norms will usually result in variations in the local tax rate.

There is therefore scope for huge variations in autonomy, even with nominally similar systems. For example, in Italy recent reforms have decentralized health care provision and (partially) finance to the regional level. The national government has defined the list of the minimum number of services to be provided by each regional system, the so-called LEA (Livelli Essenziali di Assistenza – minimum treatment levels). The list defines for each therapy group what has to be provided as a minimum, either to the entire population or to some subgroups (children, old people, means-tested people). Each region can refine and augment the list, but the treatments defined at national level have to be provided. Moreover, careful scrutiny of the Italian reforms suggests that the true autonomy of regions to vary tax rates is severely limited. Parallel reforms in Spain go much further in devolving almost all policy powers to the regions (López Casasnovas 2001). The centre's role is confined mainly to arranging redistribution of financial resources between regions. Although moving in the same direction, arrangements in the UK have in most respects not yet approached these levels of decentralization.

The impact of decentralization also depends very much on central regulations governing patients' access to health services, and how local governments reimburse providers. For example, in Italy, after a reform in 1995, each region was free to decide the level of competition between private and public providers. In some regions (Lombardy) the patient became free to choose any provider, while in others competition remains almost non-existent (Emilia Romagna). If patients are free to seek out care from any provider (public or private), and local governments must reimburse according to a national schedule of fees, then there may be little incentive for localities to develop local policies or engage in active purchasing with local providers, and limited scope for expenditure control. On the other hand, a requirement that patients use only 'preferred providers' sanctioned by the locality may have serious implications for patient choice and competition. It is noteworthy that many highly decentralized health systems (such as Canada) have a requirement that a core set of national benefits are 'portable' between jurisdictions.

Local governments experience massive variations in health needs and revenue sources. Indeed, high health needs and small tax bases often coincide. Left unattended, this situation would lead to huge variations in local services and local taxes, and a flight of mobile citizens from disadvantaged areas. Therefore, national governments invariably effect a system of grants-in-aid that often constitutes the major source of local government income. These grants are effectively a transfer from low-need, wealthy areas to high-need, poor areas, and usually seek to allow localities the opportunity to deliver some standard level of care at a standard rate of local tax and user charges (King 1984). Any system of central government transfers to localities gives the centre considerable opportunity to influence the pattern of local services. Such systems are, for example, often used by national governments as a lever for insisting on certain minimum standards in local services, or for protecting localities from certain types of risk.

THE PUBLIC ECONOMICS PERSPECTIVE
ON DECENTRALIZATION

Public economics is concerned with public goods and their financing. A public good is one that a competitive market alone cannot fully provide in line with society's wishes. We take it for granted that health and health care fall into this category. The issue we wish to address is therefore the following: given that the stewardship of the health system is a governmental responsibility when, and how, should national governments share power with more local institutions?

The principle underlying local government is that for some kinds of public good the benefits accrue to local residents, and there is, therefore, a presumption that – at least up to a point – local people should determine their nature. Economic arguments in favour of decentralizing the policymaking of public services to lower levels of government arise in a number of forms. They include the following:

- *Information*: remote national governments cannot understand all the opportunities and constraints that affect the supply of local services. They may seek to impose managerial solutions that are inappropriate for local circumstances, and strike poor bargains with providers. Equally, they may not be sensitive to variations in demand from the national norm, a particularly important consideration in health care, which is vulnerable to considerable random fluctuations in demand.
- *Preferences*: local governments can respond to local preferences and seek to design services that reflect local priorities. Local elections are the usual means of expressing such preferences, and some degree of freedom to set priorities according to local electoral choices is generally considered a pre-requisite of true local government.
- *Local coordination*: many public goods (but especially health care) require local coordination of a variety of statutory and voluntary agencies. Information limitations mean that local governments may be best placed to secure such coordination.
- *Efficiency*: because they are closer to local institutions and citizens, local managerial boards may be able to identify and root out sources of inefficiency. More generally, local people may be more prepared under decentralization to become active and encourage efficient delivery of locally-governed public services, especially if their local taxes finance the service.
- *Accountability*: the notion of accountability is often poorly

defined. However, for economists it is closely related to allocative efficiency, and reflects the idea that those who (individually or collectively) benefit from a good or service should bear the financial consequences (Barnett *et al.* 1991). Under this view, decentralization of the financing of local public goods can (if properly implemented) contribute to economic efficiency.

- *Equity*: local governments may be better placed than national governments to ensure that resources are allocated equitably within their borders.
- *Innovation*: autonomous local governments may be more willing and able to experiment with new modes of delivery.
- *Competition*: if suitable comparative information is collected and disseminated, autonomous local governments may effectively compete with each other to provide efficient and effective services through the process that has become known as 'yardstick competition' (Shleifer 1985). There may even be a 'market' in local governments offering different packages of services and different user charges and tax rates.

However, there are also economic arguments in favour of centralization, some of which directly contradict those just cited:

- *Information*: the information asymmetry between locality and centre may lead to worse outcomes under decentralization. For example, local purchasers and providers might collude to hoodwink the centre about local spending needs. More generally, local governments might act strategically in an effort to secure more than their fair share of central resources (e.g. by blaming high spending on high local needs rather than inefficiency). This phenomenon is likely to be important if central grants-in-aid depend (say) on past local expenditure levels.
- *Economies of scale*: there may be higher production, purchasing or managerial costs associated with decentralization. In particular, larger entities may be able to secure more favourable contracts with service providers. The monopsony power of the NHS as an employer of clinical staff, and its restraining influence on pay, has often been adduced as an argument in favour of central control.
- *Transaction costs*: in the UK, the managerial costs associated with small administrative units have been a persistent policy preoccupation in local government. More generally, decentralization may impose higher burdens in terms of information flows or the need for local managerial expertise to design and monitor local contracts.

- *Spillovers*: local governments may, to some extent, be inter-dependent. The services provided by one jurisdiction affect citizens from another. For example, in health care there may be public health interventions, such as childhood vaccination programmes, that will ultimately yield benefits for the whole country. Such interdependencies (or externalities) suggest some role for a national government.
- *Equity*: unfettered local government may lead to greatly varying services, standards, taxes, user charges and outcomes. These variations may compromise important equity objectives held at a national level, and so are a special class of spillover effect.
- *Macroeconomy*: the actions of local governments may collectively create important adverse macroeconomic effects. This is, for example, an argument often put forward for imposing strict borrowing controls on otherwise autonomous local governments.
- *Competition*: competition between local governments may be harmful rather than beneficial. For example, if jurisdictions compete on tax rates (because tax bases are mobile) there may be widespread under-provision of public services (Wilson 1999).

There are, of course, a number of additional reasons for seeking to decentralize services, such as promoting local democratic involvement and distributing political power in order to reduce the potential for corruption or despotism (Inman and Rubinfeld 1996). Such considerations may have important implications for efficiency and effectiveness, but in this chapter we focus only on traditional economic concerns.

Discussion of all these issues is infeasible in a single chapter. We therefore consider just three broad issues that play a central role in economic models of decentralization. The first relates to the welfare improvements associated with the increased diversity and choice that often accompanies decentralization. The second addresses the lack of information available to run services efficiently from the centre. The third concerns the potential costs that arise from fragmentation and a lack of coordination of public services.

DIVERSITY AND DECENTRALIZATION

The traditional fiscal federalism literature has focused on the extent to which decentralization allows local communities to shape local services closest to their preferences (Oates 1972). There is a general presumption that local decision-makers are better at identifying local preferences than their central counterparts, and so some form of local governance is likely to secure welfare improvements compared with a central authority.

In considering how this argument relates to health care, it is first worth noting the implications of an entirely centralized system, in which every patient's entitlement (and therefore expenditure) is explicitly defined. This assumes unambiguous information about a patient's condition and the appropriate treatment. With uniform levels of efficiency throughout the system, it might result in a system close to many systems of social security, in which a 'demand-led' national set of entitlements is carried out mechanically by local administrative offices, and is not far removed from what systems of social health insurance historically sought to secure (before recent reforms) (Normand and Busse 2002). A major implication of such a system is that it leads to an open-ended budget for the health system – demand cannot be predicted in advance, either at local or national level. It also has major managerial requirements for specifying and monitoring adherence to entitlements.

Therefore, in an attempt to secure expenditure control, many nominally centralized health systems allocate prospective budgets to local administrators, and require them (to a greater or lesser extent) to meet all local demand within that budget (Rice and Smith 2002). This approach has many virtues. It is, in practice, impossible to offer detailed epidemiological predictions of diseases and their treatment requirements. Yet, on average, the costs of delivering a given level of service to a reasonably large population can be predicted with some accuracy. Therefore, offering a global budget can often give local decision-makers an opportunity to implement the large majority of national guidelines. Within their budget, they can trade off lower than expected demand for some interventions against higher than expected demand for others, and thereby secure budgetary control to a tolerable level of accuracy.

Within such systems, central authorities often seek to circumscribe local freedom by ring-fencing some part of the local budget for specific functions, or prescribing required treatments for certain conditions (as through the National Institute for Clinical Excellence – NICE – in the UK). Such constraints circumscribe local freedom and reduce the effective degree of decentralization, but may correct for undesirable spillovers (such as failure to provide acceptable levels of care for certain chronic conditions).

Difficulties arise when the level of administrative devolution is too local, when the amount of mandatory provision is too extensive, or when the budgetary mechanism is faulty. Then, random fluctuations in demand can lead to massive overspends or underspends of budgets, and – without adequate risk-sharing arrangements – gross inequities can arise between otherwise identical patients in different localities if local decision-makers sacrifice uniformity in the interests of meeting budgets (Martin *et al.* 1998). It is for this reason that Smith (2003) advocates a range of risk-sharing arrangements when setting formulaic budgets for small administrative units such as general practices.

More decentralized systems might seek to devolve certain elements of general and fiscal policy, leading to diversity of services, taxes and user charges. The extent to which such local diversity is desired or efficient in health care – as compared to other public services – is a matter for debate. The widespread adoption of clinical guidelines and defined 'basic' packages of care suggests that many national policymakers believe that a uniform package of health care is a desirable policy objective. There is also widespread popular concern with 'postcode' rationing of health services. So the extent to which local diversity addresses policy objectives deserves careful scrutiny.

However, it is of the essence of local government that there should be some variation in levels of service and tax rates between jurisdictions. In a classic paper, Tiebout (1956) argued that citizens might 'vote with their feet' to settle in jurisdictions that provide a service mix that suits their preferences. Equally, communities might choose their mix of services deliberately to attract (or deter) certain types of citizen. A corollary of this viewpoint is that communities that fail to provide attractive services will lose mobile citizens – frequently those who provide tax revenue in excess of their demand for local public expenditure.

While Tiebout's viewpoint is deliberately extreme and provocative (and perhaps more relevant to a consumerist US setting), it nevertheless offers a great deal of food for thought when considered in relation to health care. For example, if variations in health care provision or user charges (or even local taxes) emerge, will mobile citizens move to areas offering their preferred system of health care? This is unlikely to be more than a marginal consideration so far as general acute services are concerned (although employers may take the quality of local health services into account when considering relocation decisions). However, for citizens with chronic conditions, or older people with generally high health care needs, proximity to relevant services of high quality (or low levels of user charges) might be a very important consideration when choosing where to settle. Whether the implied concentration of certain types of health care provision in certain locations leads to a welfare gain is a matter for conjecture, but local diversity is likely to benefit those who are able to move (and can therefore exercise choice) more than those who cannot.

In health care, whether local governments would seek to encourage (or deter) certain types of patient depends heavily on the finance regime (Ellis 1998). At present, geographical areas in most health systems are funded predominantly on the basis of population size, demography and general measures of socioeconomic disadvantage (Rice and Smith 2001). The extra funding for an additional citizen will therefore be a crude age-related capitation payment, albeit with some adjustment for general social conditions. Under this sort of funding arrangement, jurisdictions have a strong incentive to deter citizens they know to have health care expenditure needs in excess of the age-specific local average. That is, they may wish to deter citizens with chronic conditions, unhealthy lifestyles and generally poor health.

It is, of course, usually quite beyond the powers of local governments to explicitly refuse residence to such citizens. However, there are numerous indirect ways in which jurisdictions could signal that patients with chronic care needs are not a high priority, such as poor facilities, difficult access and even poor reported outcomes. In short, patients with long-term needs might become a very low priority in a system of competitive local governments. It is worth noting that the received wisdom in the public finance literature is that income redistribution policy should be a matter for national rather than local governments, because otherwise poorer citizens may migrate to areas with the most generous welfare regimes (Oates 1999). Analogously, if a national government is seeking to effect a 'redistribution' of health (in the form of reducing health inequalities), it is likely that this policy would be best coordinated at a national level.

A particularly interesting phenomenon arises when local governments rely on a property tax as their revenue base. Effectively, when buying a property, one secures the right to gain access to local public services as well as the intrinsic benefits of the property (and one also assumes concomitant responsibilities, in the form of local property taxes). Therefore, the property price should, in principle, partially reflect these considerations – in other words, the expected benefits and costs of local public services might be 'capitalized' into house prices. For example, there is empirical evidence that school education is, in England, a valued consideration when choosing where to live, with a large impact on house prices (Leech and Campos 2003). It is, therefore, highly likely that – if great variations in health care provision arise – similar considerations might apply.

One does not need a system of local government for the 'Tiebout effect' to arise. Indeed, the education evidence cited above arises from variations in school quality within a local government, rather than between jurisdictions. Considerable variations in service standards exist even in national government programmes, such as the NHS, and one would expect some sort of Tiebout effect to be in place already. Decentralization is merely likely to make it more pronounced if local jurisdictions introduce service variations as a matter of deliberate policy, or if variations in local taxes or user charges are permitted.

Most discussion of diversity in local government focuses on the demand side for public services. However, Besley and Ghatak (2003) present a model in which the diversity of 'missions' of local services associated with decentralization allows workers to seek out jurisdictions that most closely match their intrinsic professional motivation. Such considerations are likely to be especially important among clinicians, suggesting that there may be substantial gains to be had from a policy of health care decentralization.

INFORMATION ASYMMETRY AND DECENTRALIZATION

A central theme of fiscal federalism has always been the informational advantages enjoyed by localities to understand local demand for, and supply of, local public goods. The existence of soft, tacit local intelligence is often adduced as a fundamental reason for decentralizing decision-making. Recently, research has focused on the role of information asymmetry in determining the optimal level and nature of public service decentralization.

Seabright (1996) examines the distribution of powers between central, regional and local governments. The advantage of decentralization is that it brings electoral power closer to local people, and so may more closely align local preferences with local services. The advantage of centralization is that it permits better coordination of public goods, most notably when the choices of one locality have spillover effects for other localities. In the health domain, one particularly important spillover effect concerns the potentially negative impact of devolving choices to local government regarding various notions of equity, such as equity of health, equity of access or equity of financing.

Seabright's model presumes that governments at all levels are interested in re-election, and that the probability of re-election is determined by the level of welfare enjoyed by the population. National (or regional) governments are interested only in those lower-level areas that are marginal to their expected re-election (a sort of 'jurisdictional' median voter model). The existence of positive spillovers from one locality's services to another's welfare increases the case for centralization. However, this must be traded off against a lack of accountability in jurisdictions that are not critical to the central government's re-election.

There is an implication that aggregate spending will usually be higher under centralization, because the central government takes into account the positive spillover benefits from higher spending. Centralization also increases the willingness to transfer resources from rich to poor areas, therefore benefiting disadvantaged localities. However, Seabright's analysis suggests that centralization might benefit some localities more than others, most notably the 'pivotal' electoral battlegrounds. This prediction is borne out by research showing that, in England, national grants have been skewed to electorally important local governments (Ward and John 1999; John and Ward 2001).

Gilbert and Picard (1996) assume that central governments are less well informed than local governments about two crucial aspects of local services: local production costs and local preferences. They argue that if central government had full information on production costs, then full centralization is optimal, while the reverse is the case if the central government had full information on local preferences (including the values attached to spillovers). Ambiguity arises when (as is usually the case) there is imperfect information on both costs and preferences. If information on costs improves, then the scope for exploitation by local providers decreases, so central government is in a good position to exercise its prime role of accommodating spillover effects. If, on the other hand, information on costs is poor (or spillovers are not important), then decentralization is preferred because of local governments' better knowledge about the efficiency of local providers.

Laffont (2000) examines an important class of problem in which decentralization increases the probability of collusion between local purchasers and providers. This risk is especially important in health care, where there is an ever-present danger of local purchasers being 'captured' by powerful providers. A key element of his model is the bounded rationality of the centre in capturing and processing information about localities – in short, the information requirements of effective centralization may be costly. Once again, economic analysis offers no clear-cut policy prescription. The informational advantages of delegation have to be weighed against the potential efficiency costs of collusion. Furthermore, whether local or central governments are more vulnerable to provider 'capture' is a matter for debate.

Decentralization supported by central grants offers localities an incentive to act strategically in misrepresenting their true needs and preferences. Levaggi and Smith (1994) give an example of the nature of the game in which the locality increases its spending beyond its preferred level in order to attract higher government grants. Barrow (1986) shows how the competition between jurisdictions for a fixed central grant can induce spending in excess of efficient levels. In the same vein, Besley and Coate (forthcoming) present a model of political economy in which localities have an incentive to elect representatives with high spending preferences to national legislatures. Thus, in contrast to the view set out in the previous section, information asymmetry may lead to local expenditure that is higher than socially optimal levels.

Analyses of this sort emphasize the crucial role of information asymmetry in determining optimal structures of government. But, as Seabright (1996) argues:

> the choice between centralised and decentralised forms of government is very sensitive, not only to variable features of the particular policies in question, but to estimates of the quantitative significance of the phenomena – such as 'accountability' – that are in the nature of things very hard to quantify.

In short, while we can develop a useful framework for thinking about the decentralization problem, it is very difficult to offer concrete policy advice on optimal structures of government.

SPILLOVERS AND DECENTRALIZATION

The main role of central governments in the models discussed above is ensuring that the public services accommodate any valued spillover effects that would otherwise be ignored by local jurisdictions. Important examples of these effects can be found in any health care system, and are the reason for the generally high level of central intervention. They include:

- *Clinical training and research*: left to their own devices, localities would probably seek to 'free-ride' on the training and research provided by others, leading to chronic under-provision.
- *Public health*: given the high mobility of citizens, there is an incentive for localities to ignore actions such as health promotion that secure benefits only in the long term.
- *Inequalities*: the diversity inherent in unfettered local government, and its reluctance to address redistributional issues, may compromise nationally held equity objectives.
- *Information*: only a central authority can specify and mandate the collection of the comparative data needed for informed decision-making by politicians, managers and voters.
- *Macroeconomic factors*: the health system is a big segment of the economy with major implications for the nation's productivity. There may be a number of features of a decentralized system, such as inhibitions to labour mobility, that have adverse macro-economic consequences requiring correction by the national government.

The national government has a number of regulatory instruments available for accommodating spillovers under four broad categories: centralization of services; central rules and standards; performance reporting; and financial and non-financial incentives.

The centre can indeed internalize the spillover problem by centralizing powers. It is likely that functions such as clinical training and research should be organized directly by the centre. It is difficult to envisage any circumstances in which more oblique attempts to influence system behaviour will be as effective. However, for direct patient services there will always be a need for local organizations that purchase local services, and centralizing may merely mean the replacement of local democratic governance by a local administrator accountable to the centre.

More important than structural form are, therefore, the rules and standards imposed by the centre on local services. Whatever the governance structure, these are always likely to be extensive in health care, particularly in the domain of minimum standards of care and information provision (Petretto 2000). In the UK, standards have taken the form of guidelines, such as those promulgated by NICE and the National Service Frameworks, while in Italy and many other countries they have taken the form of a national basic package of care. Central to the effectiveness of all such instruments are the arrangements for auditing compliance, sanctions associated with departures from the standards, and the extent to which patients are empowered to ensure that standards are adhered to.

Rules concerning patients' rights can also address spillover problems. For example, a guarantee of patients' mobility can reduce inequity when the provision of hospital care is not equally distributed. For highly specialized treatments, say, patients could then move to where the intervention is supplied. Some patients (those living closer to the hospital location) will be better off than others, but the cost and quality benefits of concentrating services might outweigh the implied inequity, so long as mobility is guaranteed.

Performance reporting is becoming widespread, and one frequently-cited objective is to encourage competition and reduce disparities. However, there is an open question as to what indirect incentives might be introduced by public reporting, and the optimal deployment of comparative data remains a matter for research (Marshall *et al.* 2003). Reporting can nevertheless contribute to democratic dialogue and perhaps help the national government learn where spillovers most need attention. Certainly, the emergence of credible data from the Organization for Economic Cooperation and Development (OECD) that indicated that – relative to its international peers – the UK health system performed poorly on many aspects of health care was an important stimulus for the long-term review of the UK system undertaken by Derek Wanless (2001).

Financial incentives can take a number of forms. The traditional fiscal federalism literature considered three broad types of grant-in-aid: unconditional lump sum grants; unconditional matching grants; and conditional grants (King 1984). Each of these has very different implications for the magnitude and mix of local services and, therefore, for spillovers. Hospital systems have experimented extensively with payment mechanisms, such as fixed budgets and diagnosis-related group (DRG) funding. The former system tends to discourage treatment, while the latter can stimulate treatment in excess of optimal levels. Many academic researchers therefore advocate a 'mixed' block and DRG funding system to localities, as used in Norway (Biorn *et al.* 2003).

Levaggi and Zanola (forthcoming) examine the procedures used to distribute the total budget between competing services in a decentralized system. They find that it may be most effective to offer grants dependent on providing specific services, rather than using block grants and seeking to protect parts of the budget. In the extreme, the creation of separate local agencies for different functions may be preferred to a single local organization. There is then a trade-off with the local coordination of separate functions.

The public finance literature is concerned mainly with spillovers that lead to under-provision. However, in health care there may also be some tendency towards over-provision, or inefficient local provision. In particular, local jurisdictions often jealously guard local capital infrastructure such as hospitals, which can be considered symbols of local municipal prestige. A decentralized system might therefore lead to a system of dispersed facilities that fails to secure the economies of scale and scope offered by more concentrated patterns of infrastructure (Ferguson *et al.* 1997). The centre may have a role in ensuring that localities fully understand the potential consequences (in terms of higher costs and lower clinical quality) of maintaining a dispersed system of provision.

The 'autonomy' within which any decentralized organizations operate is highly dependent on the system of rules, standards, reporting requirements and incentives within which the centre asks them to operate. In principle, the centre probably always has enough instruments available to force localities into a particular pattern of service delivery. We would therefore argue that it should use these instruments with discretion, addressing legitimate spillover concerns, but equally ensuring that legitimate local freedoms are respected. There may be a case (in principle) for the centre subjecting every regulation it imposes to rigorous cost-benefit analysis (CBA).

CONCLUSIONS

This chapter has sought to highlight some of the important themes in the fiscal federalism literature that may be relevant to policymakers seeking to identify optimal decentralization policies in health care. We have noted the multi-dimensional nature of the concept of decentralization, and the difficulty of securing a simple definition of what it means. There are numerous economic arguments relevant to decentralization debates, but three central issues have dominated the discussion: the implications of diversity among local jurisdictions; the implications of local informational advantages; and the implications of spillover effects between jurisdictions.

Diversity among local governments, and the associated competition, can induce both beneficial and adverse behaviour. At the very least – providing the national government makes provision of comparative data mandatory – localities will be required to account to their electorate for their performance relative to their peers, through the mechanism now known as yardstick competition. The scope for competition between local jurisdictions can lead to adverse outcomes. There is a large literature that shows that the mobility of tax bases might lead to levels of local taxation that are lower than optimal, as jurisdictions 'beggar their neighbours' through tax competition. In health care, this might lead to more restricted packages of care or higher user charges than is optimal. It also creates an incentive to give services for chronically sick and elderly people a low priority. There is, therefore, an important role for national governments to assure minimum standards.

Compared to their local counterparts, national governments may suffer an informational disadvantage when purchasing services. Information asymmetries come under two broad headings: service costs and local preferences. In a service as complex as health care, it is very difficult for the centre to determine whether an apparently high level of local costs arises because of inefficiency or external demand factors. The argument for decentralization is that bringing accountability for local expenditure closer to local people will lead to increased allocative and technical efficiency.

It is not known how much variation in local preferences exists in health care. For example, it is likely that maximizing health gain is a universally held central objective of all health systems. However, it is equally reasonable to suggest that there may be considerable variation in the local weight given to issues such as access, responsiveness and equity. This being so, there is a strong case for putting local governance mechanisms in place to solicit local preferences. However, a special concern in health care is the vulnerability of the political process to 'capture' by interest groups (either patients or producers). This is an area that a vigilant central government should be alert to.

One of the main arguments for a strong central role in public services is the presence of important spillovers, when residents in one locality are affected by the nature of services in other jurisdictions. In health care there are clear reasons to believe that such spillovers are important. Variations in the availability and quality of services have obviously adverse consequences for equity. Some localities may neglect the public health and macroeconomic consequences of their services. Medical education is likely to be a national public good that would be underprovided without central coordination. These sorts of considerations provide a compelling argument for a strong central role, even in a mainly decentralized system, using minimum standards, performance reporting requirements and financial transfers.

We believe that diversity, information and spillovers are the three main considerations when discussing the optimal level of decentralization in health care. However, we noted earlier that other arguments have been adduced. Scale economies in purchasing services are often cited as an argument for centralization. However, although decentralization requires greater use of local contracting, it is difficult to identify large economies of scale to be derived from national as opposed to local purchasing of most services. Even centralized health systems such as the 'old' NHS required a local bureaucracy to purchase local services. Therefore, we think it unlikely that purchasing costs will be materially higher under decentralization.

It is also claimed that the diversity encouraged by decentralization can offer an incentive for innovation. There is scant empirical evidence to support this hypothesis, and an examination of the extremely decentralized US system offers little support for it in health care (Holahan *et al.* 2003).

One final point is that the optimal degree of decentralization is likely to be different for different health system functions. Services for primary care and chronic care may have much more scope for local discretion than (say) secondary care services, and may therefore benefit more from decentralization. Yet coordination may require that health system functions are best organized locally by a single purchaser. The optimal size and operational constraints imposed on that purchaser may therefore be something of a compromise. More generally, even if decentralization is favoured as a principle, there remains an unresolved debate about where the optimal locus of decentralization should be: for example, the Spanish region (median population several million) is very different from the Finnish municipality (median population 6000).

The appropriate level of decentralization in health care is therefore a difficult policy judgement, involving a trade-off between a number of conflicting objectives. Public economics can usefully inform the debate, but can offer no clear-cut recommendations. It is nevertheless likely that an optimal system in health care will combine a strong central role of oversight, standard-setting and information provision with a strong local role that allows local preferences to be expressed and promotes accountability of local services. It is difficult to see how this localism can be achieved in reality (rather than rhetorically) without a robust system of local democracy and some degree of financial autonomy. In their avowed aims of decentralization it will be interesting to see how far the traditionally centralized systems in countries such as the UK and Italy are prepared to embrace these principles.

DISCUSSION
Guillem López Casasnovas

The chapter examines the implications of decentralization for the equity and efficiency of public services, and adopts a neutral attitude towards decentralization. The authors suggest that economic theory is ambiguous about the merits of decentralization, a finding that is not particularly helpful for policymakers. In contrast, I should like to suggest that there is enough empirical evidence and experience to suggest that – on balance – the case for some form of fiscal and policy decentralization is strong, and can make an important contribution to improving health system performance.

A policy of decentralization is often justified on the grounds of expected efficiency gains, larger potential for innovation, better responsiveness to citizens' demands and greater social accountability. The conflict in many federal or quasi-federal systems has been the extent to which the system should limit 'regional diversity'. My view is that, to address this, a decentralized system should define a 'minimum' set of benefits to be delivered by all regions, and then allow regions to develop additional coverage at the expense of their own fiscal effort. Heterogeneous health expenditure may then result not only from differences in clinical practice, but also from different priorities in health care allocation, once regions are allowed autonomy in finance.

A fundamental difficulty in this domain is defining what is meant by decentralization. On this point the chapter is far from clear. It ranges widely across the whole gamut of decentralization, including contributions from the literature on fiscal federalism, new public management and health care payment mechanisms. Yet it does not explicitly state what is meant by decentralization. For example, does it involve political devolution (including fiscal responsibility and local political accountability), or does it refer merely to local delegation of responsibilities? Furthermore, critical to any analysis of decentralization is an understanding of the precise institutional details under consideration. For example: which powers are finally decentralized? Who decides ultimately on health policy issues? How much authority do localities have over revenue-raising capacity and spending power?

Furthermore, decentralization is not just a problem of organizational structure and institutional design. It is a multi-dimensional concept that should embrace the level of local autonomy in spending, social accountability and public responsibility. These assume very different characteristics under the four notions of decentralization: delegation, de-concentration, devolution and privatization. I shall focus on just two dimensions of decentralization: the transfer of finance powers and the transfer of policy powers.

A fundamental principle underlying public finance is that inefficiencies will arise unless – at the margin – local people bear some financial consequences for local spending decisions. However, there will always be a need for central intervention in order to preserve territorial equity. This can be done *ex-ante* (in the form of central grants-in-aid) or *ex-post* (in the form of coordination, as in Spain). However, this does not contradict the need to place at least some of the burden of local finance on a local tax base.

The issue of central coordination can be dealt with from two different perspectives. One consists of searching for formal procedures in shaping regional policies. This can be done by (i) constraining regional policy options (the so called strategy of 'less favourable output avoidance') where full autonomy might threaten the achievement of an equity-goal of the national health system, or (ii) building networks (the strategy of 'more favourable input promotion'), based on new institutions that promote regional participation in certain national policies. These formal institutions (such as the Spanish Health Inter-territorial Council) try to ensure that the legitimate views of all relevant actors on important issues inform regional policies.

A second approach to central coordination (the 'preservation of outcomes' strategy) accepts full regional autonomy, but gives the central state some paramount constitutional principles by defining certain basic notions such as the 'portability' of the entitlement of health rights between regions or overriding anti-discrimination principles, but leaving enforcement to the constitutional court.

The impact on health system effectiveness of vesting policy powers at a local level is in my view highly contingent on historical factors. One cannot predict the impact of placing new powers at a local level without knowing about the institutions and their existing competences in other spheres. In short, the behaviour of local government is path dependent, and what works in one setting may not in another.

I shall conclude with some comments on the Spanish experience. The integration of health care finance into the general financing system for all the Spanish regions has ended a political process that has been very contentious. The previous system secured little consensus among health authorities, with the only point of commonality being the claim of more resources from the central government. There have been endless disputes on the shares each region should have relative to the rest and, as a result, all health problems have been presented as due to lack of resources, with little discussion of new evidence-based policies.

Under the new arrangement, complaints about central underfinance of regional health care will have to cease. This is appropriate because, despite a common perception, Spain is not an unequal country in terms of health delivery and finance. The differences that are observed between regions in Spain relate to relatively few programmes and have little practical relevance to health status. For example, Andalusia finances certain low therapeutic value drugs from the public purse, whereas they are out of public coverage in most other regions. Only a few regions will finance sex change operations or the 'morning after' contraceptive pill.

These differences should cause little concern in equity terms as they reflect different political views on public preferences. They should be self-financed, as there seems little basis for interregional transfers to support them. Indeed, where conducted, regional opinion polls seem to favour keeping such decisions close to the citizenry affected.

Having said this, we should also recognize that we know relatively little about health differences, which derive from variations in quality of care and variations in clinical practice. It is probably not the case that there is a fundamental regional pattern in such disparities. The main equity concern probably relates to intra-regional differences rather than inter-regional differences. Those who have spoken loudest against the dangers of inter-territorial inequities have not usually made much effort to redress imbalances between local areas within the regions.

The Spanish experience shows how responsibilities in regional health provision develop as a 'learning by doing' process. An important benefit of decentralization has been the enhanced democracy and constitutional cohesion it promotes, and a consequent broader social accountability. This leads to important positive externalities. Improved health care delivery in some regions, through innovation and coverage improvements, is being extended to the other regions. Indeed, in contrast to the predictions set out by Levaggi and Smith, health care expenditure growth has been fuelled as regions seek to emulate each other, throwing into doubt the sustainability of health care funding levels.

Finally, the chapter implies that there is more scope for rent-seeking in a decentralized setting than in a centralized system. The example of the Spanish pharmaceutical industry suggests that this may not always be the case. Rather, the diversity and inter-jurisdictional competition implicit in decentralization may lead to less rather than more scope for collusion between providers and government.

The chapter nevertheless offers an excellent opportunity to understand the issues related to decentralization, not as problems, but as ways of solving some of the most important policy questions confronting national health systems.

ACKNOWLEDGEMENTS

We thank Diane Dawson and Luigi Siciliani, University of York; Richard Saltman, WHO European Observatory; and our discussant, Guillem López Casasnovas, Pompeu Fabra University, for helpful comments.

REFERENCES

Armstrong, P. and Armstrong, H. (1999) Decentralized health care in Canada, *British Medical Journal*, 318: 1201–4.
Barnett, R.R., Levaggi, R. and Smith, P. (1991) Accountability and the poll tax: the impact on local authority budgets of the reform of local government finance in England, *Financial Accountability and Management*, 7(4): 209–28.
Barrow, M. (1986) Central grants to local governments: a game theoretic approach, *Environment and Planning C: Government and Policy*, 4: 155–64.
Besley, T. and Coate, S. (forthcoming) Centralized versus decentralized provision of local public goods: a political economy approach, *Journal of Public Economics*.
Besley, T. and Ghatak, M. (2003) Incentives, choice and accountability in the provision of public services, *Oxford Review of Economic Policy*, 19(2): 235–49.

Biorn, E., Hagen, T., Iversen, T. and Magnussen, J. (2003) The effect of activity-based financing on hospital efficiency, *Health Care Management Science*, 6(4): 271–83.

Department of Health (2003) *Keeping the NHS Local – A New Direction of Travel*. London: Department of Health.

Ellis, R.P. (1998) Creaming, skimping and dumping: provider competition on the intensive and extensive margins, *Journal of Health Economics*, 17(5): 537–55.

Ferguson, B., Sheldon, T. and Posnett, J. (1997) *Concentration and Choice in Healthcare*. Edinburgh: Royal Society of Medicine Press.

Gilbert, G. and Picard, P. (1996) Incentives and optimal size of local jurisdictions, *European Economic Review*, 40(1): 19–41.

Holahan, J., Weil, A. and Wiener, J. (2003) Which way for federalism and health policy? *Health Affairs*, W3: 317–33.

Inman, R.P. and Rubinfeld, D.L. (1996) Designing tax policy in federalist economies: an overview, *Journal of Public Economics*, 60(3): 307–34.

John, P. and Ward, H. (2001) Political manipulation in a majoritarian democracy: central government target of public funds to English subnational government, in space and across time, *British Journal of Politics and International Relations*, 3(3): 308–39.

King, D. (1984) *Fiscal Tiers: The Economics of Multi-level Government*. London: Allen & Unwin.

Koivusalo, M. (1999) Decentralisation and equity of health care provision in Finland, *British Medical Journal*, 318: 1198–200.

Laffont, J.-J. (2000) *Incentives and Political Economy*. Oxford: Oxford University Press.

Lazar, H., Banting, K., Boadway, R., Cameron, D. and St-Hilaire, F. (2002) *Federal-provincial Relations and Health Care: Reconstructing the Partnership*. Ottawa: Commission on the Future of Health Care in Canada.

Leech, D. and Campos, E. (2003) Is comprehensive education really free? A case study of the effects of secondary school admission policies on house prices in one local area, *Journal of the Royal Statistical Society Series A: Statistics in Society*, 166(1): 135–54.

Levaggi, R. and Smith, P. (1994) On the intergovernmental fiscal game, *Public Finance*, 49(1): 72–86.

Levaggi, R. and Zanola, R. (forthcoming) Flypaper effect and sluggishness: evidence from regional health expenditure in Italy, *International Tax and Public Finance*.

López Casasnovas, G. (2001) *The Devolution Of Health Care to the Spanish Regions Reaches the End Point*. Barcelona: Centre for Health and Economics, Pompeu Fabreu University.

Marshall, M., Shekelle, P., Davies, H. and Smith, P. (2003) Public reporting on quality: lessons from the United States and the United Kingdom, *Health Affairs*, 22(3): 134–48.

Martin, S., Rice, N. and Smith, P.C. (1998) Risk and the general practitioner budget holder, *Social Science & Medicine*, 47(10): 1547–54.

Mills, A. (1994) Decentralization and accountability in the health sector from an international perspective: what are the choices? *Public Administration and Development*, 14: 281–92.

Normand, C. and Busse, R. (2002) Social health insurance financing, in J. Kutzin (ed.) *Funding Health Care: Options for Europe*. Buckingham: Open University Press.

Oates, W. (1972) *Fiscal Federalism*. New York: Harcourt Brace Iovanovich.

Oates, W. (1999) An essay on fiscal federalism, *Journal of Economic Literature*, 37: 1120–49.

Petretto, A. (2000) On the cost-benefit of the regionalisation of the National Health Service, *Economics of Governance*, 1: 213–32.

Pollock, A. (1999) Devolution and health: challenges for Scotland and Wales, *British Medical Journal*, 318: 1195–8.

Reverte-Cejudo, D. and Sanchez-Bayle, M. (1999) Devolving health services to Spain's autonomous regions, *British Medical Journal*, 318: 1204–5.

Rice, N. and Smith, P. (2001) Capitation and risk adjustment in health care financing: an international progress report, *Milbank Quarterly*, 79(1): 81.

Rice, N. and Smith, P. (2002) Strategic resource allocation and funding decisions, in J. Kutzin (ed.) *Funding Health Care: Options for Europe*. Buckingham: Open University Press.

Saltman, R., Bankauskaite, V. and Vrangbaek, K. (2003) *Decentralization in Health Care: Strategies and Outcomes*. Brussels: WHO European Observatory.

Seabright, P. (1996) Accountability and decentralisation in government: an incomplete contracts approach, *European Economic Review*, 40(1): 61–89.

Shleifer, A. (1985) A theory of yardstick competition, *Rand Journal of Economics*, 16(3): 319–27.

Smith, P.C. (2003) Formula funding of public services: an economic analysis, *Oxford Review of Economic Policy*, 19(2): 301–22.

Tiebout, C. (1956) A pure theory of local expenditure, *Journal of Political Economy*, 64(5): 416–24.

Wanless, D. (2001) *Securing our Future Health: Taking a Long-term View*. London: HM Treasury.

Ward, H. and John, P. (1999) Targeting benefits for electoral gain: constituency marginality and the distribution of grants to English local authorities, *Political Studies*, 47(1): 32–52.

Wilson, J.D. (1999) Theories of tax competition, *National Tax Journal*, 52(2): 269–304.

World Bank (2003) *Decentralization and Health Care*. Washington, DC: World Bank.

World Health Organization (2003) *Health Care in Transition: Country Profiles*. Copenhagen: WHO.

10

EUROPEAN INTEGRATION AND THE ECONOMICS OF HEALTH CARE

Diane Dawson, Mike Drummond and Adrian Towse[1]

INTRODUCTION

The European project has, from the beginning, been a political one. The economic benefits expected from the creation of the single market have been important (Baldwin and Venables 1995; Venables 2003), but as a means to support wider political objectives. European market integration is seen as a powerful tool for achieving political objectives. The European Union (EU) has developed legislative and judicial institutions within which promotion of an integrated market is an overriding objective rather than one to be justified solely on economic grounds. National rules and processes that impede integration are tolerated only if it can be demonstrated that they are necessary and proportionate for reasons such as the protection of public health.

In recent decades the main impediments to an integrated European economy have been non-tariff barriers – national product, service and professional standards that have the effect of protecting the domestic market, restrictive national procurement policies, and national restrictions on access of producers and consumers to other than the home market. Legislative and judicial focus has been on removing these barriers (Swann 1995). These developments have left national health care systems in an ambiguous position. The organization of health care is an area of policy reserved exclusively for the member states. However, the accumulating measures to remove barriers to movement of goods, services, capital and labour are increasingly eroding the ways in which national governments can control the health care sector.

In some circumstances member countries may feel impelled to agree common standards and mechanisms for dealing with problems that affect all countries. In the health sector we have seen harmonization of pharmaceutical licensing and approval of medical devices through the creation of the European Medicines Evaluation Agency. This is a transfer of power to regulate market entry of products from national regulators to an EU-wide regulator. Harmonizing different national regulatory regimes, each reflecting local economic and policy interests, requires the emergence of a political consensus that the benefits perceived by each country exceed the costs to the country of loss of local control. This consensus is difficult to achieve but there are identifiable areas where it may be attempted. An example for future harmonization that we consider in this chapter is that of cost-effectiveness criteria for reimbursement of pharmaceuticals.

The conflicting interests of nations may prevent the agreement needed for EU-wide harmonization in many areas of health care. However, market forces could lead towards convergence in the absence of formal harmonization. The legal framework of the EU is one that promotes development of the European single market. The principles are encapsulated in the 'four freedoms':

- freedom of movement of persons;
- freedom of movement of goods;
- freedom of movement of services;
- freedom of movement of capital.

The aim is to create a Europe-wide market and the means is the removal of impediments to competition that individual countries have erected, or may try to erect, to protect local markets. Recent judgements of the European Court of Justice (ECJ), combined with policy changes being introduced piecemeal by member states, are opening up new opportunities for patients, and for companies providing health care services across borders.

WHY REGULATE, AND WHERE?

Regulation has the traditional functions of overcoming market failure due to:

- asymmetric information;
- externalities;
- market power.

Gatsios and Seabright (1989) examine conditions under which it is in the interests of an individual country to delegate national regulatory powers to a single EU regulator. If we focus on the health care sector, these considerations can be grouped under the headings of:

- cost;
- credibility;
- coordination.

Health technology licensing and assessments of cost-effectiveness are designed to deal with problems of asymmetric information. The question is whether these problems may be more effectively dealt with at the EU level. Aside from infectious diseases, there are few externalities that would require harmonization of benefit packages across Europe. The one exception would appear to be the overuse, in some European countries, of antibiotics that may create many new resistant bacteria that could have community-wide public health and cost consequences (Maynard 2002/3). National regulation of market power has usually been directed at inhibiting attempts by companies to reduce competition (anti-trust or anti-cartel legislation). However, governments also use their powers to promote the interests of particular domestic industries. To date, the main European concern with market power in health care has been the power of governments to erect discriminatory barriers, protecting local producers in areas like public procurement, market entry and the movement of patients. ECJ decisions on restrictions by national governments regarding the marketing of generic drugs and parallel imports of pharmaceuticals have reduced national barriers and increased intra-community trade.

HARMONIZATION: OPPORTUNITIES AND CONSTRAINTS

The impact on health care of EU harmonization can be significant. The most obvious example is the European Working Time Directive (EWTD) and the consequences for staffing of hospitals. The need to change the working patterns of junior doctors is leading to significant changes in service delivery at small- and medium-sized hospitals.

Another example is the harmonization of arrangements for market approval (i.e. licensing) of new pharmaceuticals and medical devices through the establishment of the European Medicines Evaluation Agency (EMEA). In this case, member states have agreed on a common set of procedures for assessing the efficacy, safety and quality of manufactured drugs. Once approved by the EMEA, the products can be sold throughout the EU.

Harmonization of drug licensing has highlighted an even greater problem facing member states: how to decide on the products that will be included in a benefit package and the price that will be paid for new drugs. There is a fair degree of agreement that existing systems are not working well (Garrison and Towse 2003). Maynard (2002/3) has called for harmonization: 'The ideal institution for Europe would be a Euro-NICE'.[2]

Harmonization of reimbursement and pricing for health technologies

When considering what economic issues are relevant to an analysis of whether it may be desirable to harmonize reimbursement and pricing decisions within a Euro-NICE, a useful starting point is to consider the key characteristics of an efficient system, then look at reasons for failure to achieve efficiency and, finally, to consider the contribution harmonization could make to reducing inefficiency.

In Figure 10.1a we consider the position of an individual member state. Only cost-effective treatments are offered. Interventions reimbursed under the national health insurance system are ranked by expected equity weighted quality-adjusted life years (QALYs) per € (000). This is simply the inverse of the familiar cost per QALY used in cost-effectiveness studies. The most cost-effective treatments have priority so that, as the health care budget increases, more patients have access to treatments with lower expected benefits per €. For a given set of medical technologies, the expected relationship between the size of the health care budget and the cost-effectiveness of the marginal treatment provided is reflected in the curve UK.[3] UK is the frontier for an efficient system, while the current size of the budget and implied cost-effectiveness threshold reflects society's willingness to pay for health care at the margin.[4] In Figure 10.1a the total available budget is C, with an implied incremental QALY gain for the last € spent of D.

In Figure 10.1b we consider the impact of introducing a new therapy in one country. When a new therapy appears on the market, it is evaluated by the local NICE in terms of expected cost-effectiveness and budgetary impact. Where the expected equity weighted outcome

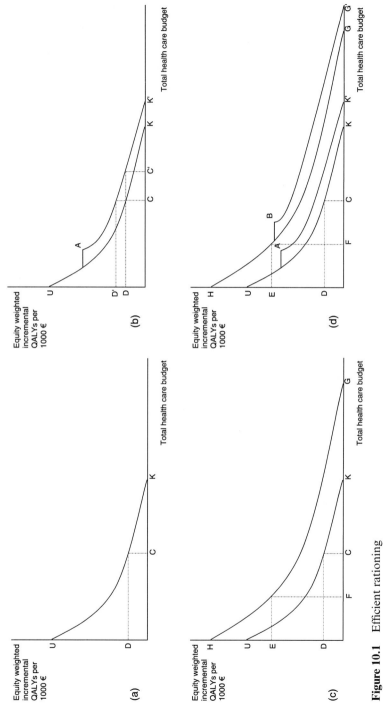

Figure 10.1 Efficient rationing

per € is greater than zero, the curve UK shifts outward to UAK′. The point at which the new therapy enters the frontier is determined by the expected cost-effectiveness relative to other therapies. If the budget remains constant at C, the implied marginal QALY gain per € rises to D′. Introduction of the new therapy displaces existing marginal treatments. If the regulator maintains the cost-effectiveness threshold at D, total health care expenditure must rise to C′.

Arguments for harmonization require analysis of the circumstances of more than one country. In Figure 10.1c we compare the efficient system frontiers of two member states for a given set of medical technologies. The frontier for the second country, HG, may differ from that of UK for several reasons. The clinical effectiveness of interventions is likely to be similar across countries (Drummond and Pang 2001) but cost-effectiveness and budgetary impact may differ due to differences in:

- the equity weights placed on QALYs (age, gender, social class);
- the real cost of delivering treatment (factor prices, clinical practice, capacity);[5]
- the relative size of the patient groups requiring different treatments (respiratory disease v. heart disease).

The case illustrated is where the cost of treatment is systematically lower in country HG than in UK (hence the HG frontier lies outside the UK frontier). For any given size of the health care budget, the marginal € purchases more QALYs in HG than in UK. HG also has a lower total expenditure on health care with a budget of F and implied (inverse) cost-effectiveness threshold E. The order of magnitude of the difference between E and D may be inferred from the suggestion that the cost-effectiveness threshold in HG (i.e. Hungary) may be around €13,000, while it is around €50,000 in the UK (i.e. in the United Kingdom (Szende *et al.* 2002). In Figure 10.1c this would imply incremental QALYs per € (000) of 0.08 at E and 0.02 at D. The two frontiers might approximate to those of a relatively poor country and a relative wealthy country within the EU.

In Figure 10.1d we consider the positions of both countries when a new therapy is introduced. After cost-effectiveness analysis (CEA) by the independent NICE of each country and, given the national budget constraints, UK would want to include the product in the package of services provided, but HG would not. Where each individual country is internally efficient, societal willingness to pay differs and there are no externalities, there would be no case on efficiency grounds to delegate national regulatory functions to a Euro-NICE and no case for a uniform reimbursement decision. HG should not be required to include the new therapy and UK should not be prevented from including it in the benefit package. Note that this conclusion holds even though expected QALYs per € from the new therapy appear to be higher in HG than in UK.

However, we know that the reimbursement decisions in member countries are not efficient. In all cases the actual frontier lies within the efficient system frontier. The issue is therefore whether any moves toward harmonization may help to reduce existing national inefficiencies relative to no harmonization. Considering the Gatsios and Seabright criteria, two elements appear relevant.

First, consider the *cost* and capacity to undertake thorough cost-effectiveness evaluations. EU member states vary in their capacity to undertake high-quality evaluation and modelling of new interventions. This problem has been exacerbated by the entry of the east European countries in 2004 (Szende *et al.* 2002). As with the EMEA, there could be benefits in pooling expertise and sharing the costs of producing what is a public good (Rehnberg 2002). The quality of information provided would be an improvement for relatively poor countries and, if there are economies of scale, more interventions may be evaluated than even wealthy countries working independently could finance. It is worth noting that even in the UK there is an annual limit on the number of evaluations that NICE can perform. Most European countries focus scarce evaluation resources on new products, but we know that system-wide efficiency also requires that we evaluate old products that may not be cost-effective, so that they can be excluded from the benefit package. If avoiding duplication of effort at the national level allowed an expansion in the number of procedures evaluated, all countries could increase the rate at which they identified inefficient procedures and, if these were removed from the package, the actual frontier could be shifted outward toward the efficient system frontier. To secure these gains would not require the full 'Maynard' Euro-NICE, but a Euro-almost-NICE. If it is true that clinical effectiveness does not vary significantly by country but costs do, presentation of results over a range of cost assumptions would be required. This would improve the ability of each member state to relate expected outcomes to local cost conditions but would not impose a Europe-wide cost-effectiveness threshold.

Second, there is the issue of *credibility*. All regulators are subject to the risk of regulatory capture. Most governments find the local interests of clinicians, patient advocates, providers and pharmaceutical companies difficult to control. Given national differences in at least the first three groups, a Euro-NICE that selected and evaluated interventions may be less subject to regulatory capture than national regulators. With the exception of pharmaceutical companies, the other interest groups are likely to be more fragmented at the European level than at the national level. If this is correct, some delegation of national regulation may be to the benefit of all member states. Where risks of regulatory capture are reduced, the actual frontier for each country would shift outward toward the efficient system frontier.

An issue of fundamental importance is whether the introduction of a Euro-NICE would create a more effective counterbalance to the market power of the pharmaceutical industry than a set of independent national regulators (Cookson and Hutton 2003). This is an important strand of the Maynard argument, and could be considered under the Gatsios and Seabright heading of *coordination*. Maynard's case for harmonization would be in stark contrast to that usually put forward for the creation of a single market. The standard economic analysis is that a single market produces welfare gains by increasing the diversity of products available and/or realizing economies of scale (Nerb 1988; Gatsios and Seabright 1989). EMEA has been seen as a means of strengthening the competitive position of the pharmaceutical industry. An effective Euro-NICE might reduce market opportunities for the industry, and reduce the diversity of products reimbursed, in the interest of securing welfare gains for the population of Europe.

Methodological issues in harmonization of cost-effectiveness studies

Harmonization in drug licensing arrangements was greatly aided by the fact that there are standardized approaches for conducting efficacy studies (i.e. randomized controlled trials) and that the results of such studies can often be generalized (i.e. the efficacy of the drug in a given patient group is likely to be similar in one EU country compared with another).

As mentioned above, the same assumption about the generalizability of cost-effectiveness results does not hold. Factors known to vary from country to country are likely to impact upon the cost-effectiveness of health care interventions. Even if we accept that, owing to differences in the willingness to pay for QALYs among EU countries, there is no case for a uniform reimbursement decision, the more limited role of a Euro-almost-NICE (the production of high-quality cost-effectiveness evidence) would pose a number of methodological challenges.

The challenges are less complex in the case of modelling studies, since the approach in these economic evaluations is to populate the model with data relevant to the decision-making problem at hand. In this case the challenge would be to locate the best available data for the various countries of the EU. In most situations it would be possible to use the same efficacy data for all countries, alongside varying data (by country) for patterns of resource use, prices and health state valuations.

Several researchers have explored approaches for analysing multi-national economic clinical trials (Drummond and Pang 2001), the most promising of which is multi-level modelling (Manca *et al.* in press). Here the hierarchical nature of the data is recognized, with patients being nested within clinical centres which themselves are nested within countries. It is then possible to produce country-specific (indeed centre-specific) estimates of cost-effectiveness from a multi-national trial. However, these approaches require large amounts of data and considerable planning is required to undertake the appropriate data collection in the various centres and countries. Therefore, it would make sense for such studies to be planned and executed as a single entity, although this would not necessarily need to be within a central European agency.

Despite the recent progress in developing methods for the analysis of multi-national economic clinical trials, several challenges remain. These include: (i) generating cost-effectiveness estimates for countries not included in the trial; and (ii) devising standardized costing procedures given the wide variety of accountancy practices in European health care systems. Whether the potential benefits of harmonizing procedures for conducting cost and cost-effectiveness analysis (CEA) can be realized depends on progress in dealing with many of the methodological issues raised.

Defining the health benefit package

Whether reimbursement and pricing decisions are made on the national or European level, the definition of the health benefit package is a central component of health care financing. A full Euro-NICE would, over time, lead to greater uniformity in the benefit package across Europe. However, it is difficult to see why this should be an objective of the emerging regulatory framework.

Differences in individual preferences and social preferences reflected (imperfectly) in the scope of public services are not indicators of market failure. There is a fundamental distinction between reserving the right of nation states to define the benefits to which their residents are entitled through the social security system and ensuring that, once defined, there are no disproportionate obstacles to competition between European providers in the supply of these services.

Until the Smits-Peerbooms decision (European Court of Justice 2001a) the ECJ had not directly addressed the issue of the treatments to which a patient is entitled in countries that provide benefits-in-kind health services. In all EU countries there has always been the power to exclude treatments from the national health care package.[6] As long as the reasons for limiting the health care package are published, transparent and non-discriminatory, the ECJ has upheld these exclusions. However, in most benefit-in-kind systems, the effective benefit package is defined implicitly and constantly changes with local medical practice. In the Netherlands patients are entitled to medically necessary treatment that is considered 'normal in professional circles'. The ECJ considered whether this way of defining the benefit package could be used as a covert way of reducing competition between providers.

The Smits-Peerbooms cases concerned patients with conditions clearly covered by the Dutch health care system (Parkinson's disease and coma following a traffic accident), but each patient requested access to specific therapies that are available in other EU countries, but not in the Netherlands. In Mrs Smits case, her sickness fund argued that the specific clinical method requested by the patient (available in Germany) was not regarded as normal treatment within the relevant Dutch professional circles and therefore was not one of the benefits covered by the fund (para. 29). In the Peerbooms case the patient's consultant requested a particular neurological treatment, available in Austria but considered experimental in the Netherlands. A Dutch patient would have to be enrolled in the domestic trial to receive the treatment, but the trial was restricted to patients under the age of 25. Mr Peerbooms was 36 and therefore not eligible for the trial. The sickness fund argued that the treatment was therefore not part of the benefits package.

The ECJ ruled that 'normal' treatment could not be defined solely by reference to professional practice in the Netherlands, but must reflect international medical evidence: 'The requirement that the treatment must be regarded as "normal" is construed to the effect that authorisation cannot be refused on that ground where it appears that the treatment concerned is sufficiently tried and tested by international medical science' (para. 108).

The two Dutch patients lost their cases, but the requirement that 'normal' treatment be defined with reference to the international scientific literature is now embedded in European case law. This can have important implications for future determination of benefit packages within European countries.

Many commentators expect there to be a significant increase in the number of patients wishing to exercise some choice over the type of treatment they receive. This will be particularly important for patients with chronic conditions and preferences over the patient pathway. All member states will have to deal with this problem. Would a Euro-NICE with a reputation for high-quality review of the evidence be viewed as an independent reference point for member countries in dealing with questions of whether various treatments are, or are not, 'sufficiently tried and tested by international medical science', and, therefore, potentially part of the implicit benefit package? Cost-effectiveness thresholds are likely to continue to vary between countries, but it would be surprising if regular European reviews of the medical evidence for different therapies did not lead to some convergence of the implicit benefit package.

A Euro-almost-NICE would provide member states with evaluations based on a range of cost assumptions, and would make it easier for each country to arrive at decisions that may be relatively efficient in local circumstances. Information generated by these studies could make national differences in the costs of delivering particular interventions more transparent. That information could benefit local regulators. It could also have the important consequence of beginning to move European policy for health technologies out of the clutches of EU industrial policy, where the aim is to promote the interests of the industry, and into the health policy domain, where the objective is to deliver more efficient health care.

MARKET FORCES, DOMESTIC REFORM AND THE ECJ

To date EU governments have been very reluctant to agree harmonization measures for the health care sector, and anything approaching a Euro-NICE is a distant prospect. However, the failure to agree a framework that sets out clear objectives for the development of health care in Europe is proving to be problematic. A succession of decisions by the ECJ is opening health care to market forces. The cumulative impact of these decisions could undermine the national sovereignty over health care that governments want to protect.

The role of the ECJ is to ensure that community law is interpreted and applied consistently in member states. This law is embedded in the Treaty of the community and in secondary legislation. Promotion of the internal market and the principles of the 'four freedoms' form part of the treaty. Equivalent principles for the objectives and principles of health care within Europe are absent. As a result of this asymmetry, health care policies of member countries that appear to restrict choice and competition are judged by the objectives of the market, rather than principles that reflect the objectives of European health care. It has been suggested that the Treaty should set out, for health care, principles equivalent to those for the single market. For health these could constitute universality, solidarity and equity (Berman 2002/3). To date, the ECJ has allowed, as justification for some restrictions on market freedom, potentially serious damage to the planning and financial viability of a universal health care system (see below).

The UK, a country that has consistently opposed cases brought before the ECJ by plaintiffs objecting to national restrictions on their right to use cross-border health care, is introducing a number of changes to the National Health Service (NHS) that *increase* the likelihood that the ECJ will find fewer arguments to support national restrictions. On balance this will increase the case for a more open European market. When we combine domestic policy changes with the orientation of the ECJ, the scene is set for greater influence of the European market on the NHS.

Emerging market forces

To illustrate the way a country's local policy decisions can have (unintended) Europe-wide implications, we consider a few recent changes to the NHS. Other EU countries are pursuing variations on some of these policies and the issues are not parochial. The NHS changes of most relevance in this context are the introduction of a National Tariff, patient choice and expansion of providers to include the UK private sector as well as international providers.

The National Tariff

When supporting the case against Kholl and Decker (European Court of Justice 1998), the UK and other governments argued that benefit-in-kind systems of health care had no prices and therefore no rates relevant to reimbursement of services obtained outside the NHS. However, the government is in the process of introducing fixed prices for procedures delivered to NHS patients (Department of Health 2003). The National Tariff will apply to services purchased from NHS Trusts, Foundation Hospitals, the UK private sector and overseas providers. The introduction of a National Tariff may have important implications for the market. The ECJ has upheld the right of governments to fix maximum prices for health care services, but it will be interesting to observe how it responds to denial of the right to compete by offering lower prices.

Patient choice

Expanding patient choice is now a policy objective of the NHS (Department of Health 2002). Of particular importance will be the ability to purchase diagnostic services and other ambulatory care from a wider range of suppliers. From the limited evidence available, it is apparent that patients are reluctant to travel for in-patient treatment. However, it is not clear to what extent the evidence reflects consumer preferences or the tendency of local clinicians to discourage, or not cooperate with, choice.[7] Where demand reflects strong locational preferences we usually observe suppliers moving into the market area of consumers, rather than consumers moving to suppliers. However, there may be a higher proportion of patients willing to travel for diagnostic services. Reduced waiting time for diagnostic treatment has two benefits for patients. First, it reduces the anxiety of not knowing the severity of symptoms and, second, it can be a means of moving up the waiting list when tests indicate the condition is serious. We would expect that a higher proportion of patients would be willing to travel for ambulatory care than for in-patient treatment, and changes in medical practice are increasing the substitution of ambulatory care for in-patient treatment. All the high profile ECJ decisions have concerned the right of national governments to restrict patient choice of cross-border care.

Unbundling of hospital services and new entry

Once prices have been set for individual diagnostic tests, procedures, accident and emergency (A&E) attendances etc. the question arises as to whether suppliers have an incentive to 'unbundle' traditional hospital procedures and invest in units that specialize in one area of activity. Units that specialize in diagnostic testing are found in several countries. In the USA there are private companies that specialize in free-standing A&E units. A limited private sector unit has recently opened in England (Casualty Plus). England is encouraging both private and public sector companies to establish Diagnostic and Treatment Centres (DTCs) that specialize in particular procedures (ophthalmology, orthopedics etc.). The Department of Health has recently selected firms from the USA, South Africa and Canada as preferred bidders for private sector DTCs that will be awarded secure NHS contracts (*Healthcare Market News* 2003).

The capital investment required for these specialist units is considerably below that for an integrated hospital. Barriers to entry should, therefore, be lowered. Certainly the call for tenders for new DTCs, and the recent history of Private Finance Initiative (PFI) consortia and privatized utilities suggests little reluctance from European and other international companies to invest in UK firms delivering public services.

Planning capacity

What are to be the controls on new entry? In the past, the Department of Health has exercised no control over entry of private sector health care providers, while exercising tight control over public sector providers. It would appear that a new policy is now emerging, influencing new private sector entry by offering low-risk contracts to preferred providers. Providers who wish to enter the higher risk, uncontracted market are still free to do so.

The situation in England is in stark contrast to that in France. The French health care planning system covers *all providers*, be they public, private not-for-profit or private for-profit. Planned new investment in hospital capacity or major diagnostic equipment (e.g. scanners) must obtain central approval. Once 'planning permission' is given, companies seek public or private funding depending on the nature of the organization.

The 'planning' system obviously makes an important difference to the operation of the market. 'Free entry' could be restricted to the equivalent of bidding for 'slots' at major airports, where a government controls the number and size of the airports. If firms 'own' their slots, takeover and merger is a mechanism for reallocating slots. If property rights over the slots are retained by the regulator, greater control can be exercised over new entrants. There could be challenges to restrictions on new entry. This is more likely to come from the expansion of the World Trade Organization (WTO) into the sphere of health services than current pressures within the EU. While the UK may be most vulnerable to these developments, the consequences would be felt throughout Europe.

If member states are unable to agree principles for the health care sector and the single market (re. industrial) agenda continues to impinge on health care, will our economic models tell us anything about how the market may develop (Church and Ware 2000)? Many of the changes outlined in this section have implications for new entry. Health care is classically a market with product differentiation, mainly by location but also by quality and type of product. The most appropriate models are the address models that have been developed from the work of Hotelling (1929).

Contracting and control of capacity

Those recent judgements of the ECJ causing the most consternation in national health ministries have nominally been about the rights of patients wishing to obtain treatment, paid for by their health insurance scheme, from providers in other EU countries with which the insurer did not have contracts. In the process of arriving at decisions in these particular cases, the ECJ has pronounced on a number of issues of wider significance for the organization of health care. For the first time, some of these arguments have appeared in an English High Court judgement (High Court of Justice Queen's Bench Division 2002) with an interpretation that raises important economic issues.

The ECJ has ruled that when governments restrict the right of a patient to obtain treatment, covered by the national health care system, from another European supplier, there is a prima facie restriction on the freedom to provide services in the single market. The defendants in these cases (sickness funds) have, with the support of the UK, argued that restricting freedom of choice to providers with which the fund has contracts is necessary in order to plan and control hospital capacity. This is seen as necessary to ensure the obligation under the Treaty of providing 'a high level of health protection' (Article 152).

To date, the ECJ has agreed (European Court of Justice 2001a: paras 76–9). In the Smits-Peerbooms case it argued that, in contrast to ambulatory services:

> medical services provided in a hospital take place within an infrastructure with, undoubtedly, certain very distinct character-

istics. It is thus well known that the number of hospitals, their geographical distribution, the mode of their organisation and the equipment with which they are provided, and even the nature of the medical services which they are able to offer, are all matters for which planning must be possible. This kind of planning therefore broadly meets a variety of concerns; it seeks to achieve the aim of ensuring that there is sufficient and permanent access to a balanced range of high-quality hospital treatment in the State concerned. It also assists in meeting a desire to control costs and to prevent, as far as possible, any wastage of financial, technical and human resources. It is generally recognized that the hospital care sector generates considerable costs and must satisfy increasing needs, while the financial resources which may be made available for health care are not unlimited, whatever the mode of funding applied.

An important caveat has been applied to this justification: the treatment to which the patient is entitled must be available from a contracted provider 'without undue delay'.

In all judgements the ECJ has repeated the long-standing principle that in awarding contracts there must be no discrimination against providers from other European countries. When, in 2001, the Department of Health denied the right of health authorities and Primary Care Trusts (PCTs) to contract with other European hospitals, but encouraged contracting with UK private sector hospitals, it was in clear violation of EU law. This was technically rectified when, for a brief time in 2002–3, the Department entered into a few limited contracts with other EU hospitals, but it would appear that very few patients are now offered this option. Where a health care system makes use of non-contracted providers, national providers must not be given preference over other EU providers. The UK has been in violation of this condition, in that it regularly makes use of non-contracted UK private sector providers, while restricting the use patients can make of non-contracted EU providers.

Watts v. Bedford PCT and the Secretary of State for Health

In October 2003 Mr Justice Mumby delivered his High Court judgement in the case of *Watts* v. *Bedford PCT and the Secretary of State for Health*. Mrs Watts was diagnosed as having osteoarthritis in both hips. The consultant wrote that she had severe bilateral hip pain and severe deterioration in mobility and had to use two walking sticks 'to mobilize'. The waiting time would be approximately one year and, given the severity of other patients on his waiting list, there was no case to treat her as requiring more urgent treatment. Mrs Watts applied to her PCT for authorization (E112) to be treated abroad, where the procedure would be carried out in two weeks, at a price less than the NHS average reference cost (now National Tariff) and considerably less than the price the NHS pays UK private providers for this procedure. Her request was turned down on the grounds that treatment within one year would meet NHS waiting time targets and therefore did not constitute 'undue delay'. After initiation of litigation and continued approaches to the PCT and Department of Health, Mrs Watts was reassessed as having deteriorated sufficiently to be given a three- to four-month wait. In the meantime she had arranged for treatment in France. The High Court ruled that while she was right, and the PCT and Secretary of State had acted unlawfully in denying authorization for treatment abroad, the revised waiting time did not constitute 'undue delay' and, therefore, she was not entitled to reimbursement of the cost of her treatment in France.

As in all these cases, it is not the final outcome for the plaintiff, but the principles elucidated that will affect future actions. The English judge concurred with earlier ECJ judgements that 'It is not clear from the arguments submitted to the ECJ that such waiting times are necessary for the purpose of safeguarding the protection of public health. On the contrary, a waiting time which is too long or abnormal would be more likely to restrict access to balanced, high quality hospital care' (European Court of Justice 2001a: para. 144). If existing capacity constraints are not arguments accepted by the ECJ for refusing choice of a non-contracted provider, defendants (and the UK government) had argued that authorizing treatment in another member state would undermine the financial balance of the domestic health care system. The ECJ stated that this would be a justification for restricting choice if it would lead to financial wastage resulting from hospital under-utilization (para. 143), but *not* if existing capacity continued to be fully utilized.

The High Court judgement was stark. The fact that the UK government had restricted capacity to levels that could not deliver treatments which patients were entitled to, under the implicit benefit package, and therefore needed to manage that restricted capacity, was not relevant to the determination of undue delay and the right of patients to seek funded treatment elsewhere. While the judge did not use the term, there was an implicit questioning of national autonomy in deciding social (or government) willingness to pay, and the implied scope of entitlements of individuals in European health care systems.

The ECJ seemed to be implying that if the finance and organization of health care in the UK, or any other country, leads to patients with the clinical condition of Mrs Watts waiting 12 months for treatment, then the health care system is not meeting its obligation under Article 152 to provide high-quality health protection. The fact that the UK is currently investing in more capacity, in the hope of avoiding this kind of delay in the near future, is not relevant. A future government could again restrict funding for the NHS and these problems would re-emerge. The issue, therefore, remains whether European jurisprudence will question the right of member states to restrict access to the implicit benefits package solely on the grounds of domestic economic policy.

If waiting time, part of the implicit benefit package, is questioned by the ECJ, what other elements of the benefit package may be subject to review through ECJ judgements? NICE guidance frequently seeks to place restrictions on individuals' capacity to seek care. For example, it is quite common for NICE to recommend that a health technology only be made available for individuals meeting certain clinical criteria. In some cases, these relate to progression of disease and the seriousness of the patient's condition (e.g. NICE argued that photodynamic therapy for macular degeneration should only be given when the patient's eyesight had deteriorated to a certain degree). At present it is not clear whether the courts will seek to question the level at which these restrictions are placed.

Patient choice, reimbursement and EU enlargement

The ECJ is becoming involved in defining the benefit packages of member states. This then requires evidence-based treatment and a possible future definition of what constitutes undue delay.

ECJ judgements have resulted in some confusion as to the basis for reimbursing treatment that patients from one member state receive in another. This increases the uncertainty of budget-holders in all countries, but could be a particularly serious problem with enlargement. Expansion of the EU from the existing 15 members to 25 has brought 10 relatively poorer countries into the EU. To what extent will patients from Poland or Hungary now seek treatment in Germany or France, where the availability and cost of treatment is greater than in the home country? Under the Article 22 arrangements for prior authorization (E112), the cost of treatment was reimbursed on the basis of the prices prevailing in the country of treatment. The Kohl and Decker decisions opened the possibility of reimbursement at the tariffs prevailing in the country of residence. The decision in the Vanbraekel case (European Court of Justice 2001b) stated that if the reimbursement based on home tariffs was less than that based on the country of treatment, there would be an impediment to the free movement of services within the single market.

This is a classic example of why EU countries need to agree a framework for health services that supports health service objectives, rather than the objectives of the single market. Budgets for health care in the new member states could be put under pressure if patients exercise choice and reimbursement must be at west European rates. If political agreement could be reached whereby reimbursement would, in all cases, be at the tariff of the home country, patient choice need not result in a significant depletion of national health care budgets. How the European health care market develops depends on whether governments decide to agree policies, or to leave these issues to the courts.

CONCLUSIONS

In this chapter we have tried to look forward to a few of the economic issues likely to be on the agenda of economists working in the field of health care as European integration progresses. The case for harmonization is weak, but the alternative may be worse, as the rules of the single market impinge on the development of national health care systems.

The single market agenda reflects a political imperative and a questionable economic model. At one extreme, emergence of a Euro-NICE, a single market for pharmaceuticals and a common benefit package would impose significant costs on the poor and middle-income members of the EU. It has been suggested that these developments would require the creation of a mechanism for major fiscal redistribution along the lines of the Common Agricultural Policy in order to prevent the single market from increasing inequality in access to health care.

If health economists are to make a contribution to the direction of change in Europe, it is essential that they address key issues. The economics of the single market rests on assumptions that increased competition and product diversity are welfare enhancing. These are questionable in the health care sector. Consumers of health care are insured and finance is, in all west European countries, primarily from general taxation or (in effect) earmarked taxes. Treatment protocols and cost-effectiveness hurdles seek to reduce product diversity and choice on efficiency grounds. Some new thinking on the welfare economics of market integration is needed if we are to apply it to health care.

In Europe the concept of 'solidarity' has placed primacy on equity in access to health care, not competition between different benefit packages. Solidarity is compatible with competition in supply of services, but unless we develop a better understanding of how competition in supply, and the regulation of competition, impinges on equity of access, there is a danger that the competition agenda of the single market will inadvertently erode equity of access.

For the last 70 years, since the seminal work of Ramsey on efficient pricing, economists have recognized that there are circumstances under which welfare can be enhanced by the adoption of multiple prices rather than a single market price. This is particularly important in health care, but has received little attention in the present EU debate as the objective of a single market has intruded into pricing of pharmaceuticals and health care services.

It is a rich agenda not only for research but also for active involvement of health economists in the EU policy debate.

APPENDIX

The 'efficient' frontier used in Figure 10.1 assumes only cost-effective therapies are offered. It illustrates how the marginal health gain purchased declines with the size of the health care budget. The information required to estimate the frontier is outlined in Table 10.1. In theory, an organization like NICE is expected to collect information for columns a, b, c, e and f. If we have b and c, we can calculate d and then rank therapies by QALYs per €(000). Starting with the most cost-effective therapies, estimates of the cost per patient episode (c) times the expected number of patients (e) gives the expected total budgetary impact of the therapy (f). The rate at which each therapy absorbs the health care budget (g) can then be plotted against expected incremental health gain (d).

Figure 10.2 is a histogram presentation of the relevant data. For Figure 10.1, in the text, it has been smoothed to a curve. To illustrate the effect of introducing a new product, we take the example of condition D that had absorbed a small share of the budget. The new product promises a higher health gain per € than the existing treatment and a larger number of patients may benefit. In Figure 10.3 this results in displacement of all therapies from C onwards.

Table 10.1 Data Required for Efficient Rationing

Procedure/patient characteristics (a)	Expected health gain (QALYs or other measure) (b)	Expected cost per patient episode (€) (c)	Expected health gain per €000 (d)	Expected number of patients to be treated (e)	Expected total cost (€m) (f)	Cumulative total expenditure (€m) (g)
A						
B						
C						
D						
E						
F						

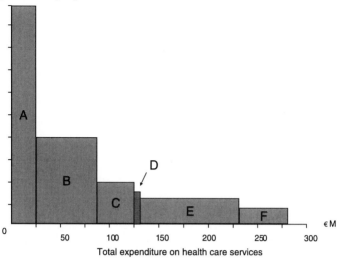

Expected health gain per € 000

Figure 10.2   Ranking of cost-effective treatments by health gain and total expenditure

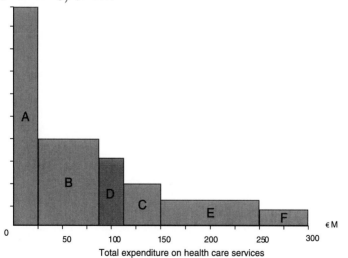
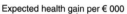

Expected health gain per € 000

Figure 10.3   Impact of a new product on ranking of cost-effective treatments

ACKNOWLEDGEMENTS

Development of the graphical presentation of the cost per QALY budget impact frontier benefited from discussions with Alan Williams. Translation of sketches into Figure 10.1a–d is due to the skill of Andrew Street.

NOTES

1   Adrian Towse acted as discussant for a previous version of this chapter and was added as an author to the updated version, at the authors' request.
2   NICE is the acronym for the National Institute for Clinical Excellence, established by the UK government to evaluate the cost-effectiveness and budgetary impact of drugs, surgical procedures and other medical treatments. NICE recommends to the government whether a therapy should be available to National Health Service (NHS) patients. The government then decides whether to accept the recommendation. If the guidance is accepted, purchasers must fund the therapy but the guidance is not binding on clinicians.
3   Information required to construct curve UK is given in the appendix.
4   We are well aware of the arguments against a single cost-effectiveness 'threshold'. Rather, our argument only requires that an individual member state has the means to rank treatments based on the opportunity cost of generating an equity-weighted QALY.
5   Differences in capacity are efficient if they reflect differences in social willingness to pay for waiting time. Capacity costs will be inefficient if they reflect market and regulatory failures that result in excess capacity greater than that implied by willingness to pay for waiting time.
6   In the UK this requires specification in Schedules 10 or 11 of the National Health Service (NHS) (General Medical Services) Regulations 1992.
7   In England there are a few discrete choice experiments in the progress of analysis that may shed some light on this issue.

REFERENCES

Baldwin, R.E. and Venables, A.J. (1995) Regional economic integration, in G. Grossman and K. Rogoff (eds) *Handbook of International Economics Volume III*, pp. 1597–644. Amsterdam: Elsevier Science.

Berman, P.C. (2002/3) The EU health and Article 152: present imperfect, future perfect? *Eurohealth*, 8(5): 4–7.

Church, J. and Ware, R. (2000) Product differentiation, in J. Church and R. Ware (eds) *Industrial Organisation: A Strategic Approach*, pp. 367–421. Maidenhead: McGraw-Hill.

Cookson, R. and Hutton, J. (2003) Regulating the economic evaluation of pharmaceuticals and medical devices: a European perspective, *Health Policy*, 63: 167–78.

Department of Health (2002) *Delivering the NHS Plan: Next Steps on Investment, Next Steps on Reform*. London: DoH.

Department of Health (2003) *Payment by Results: Consultation-preparing for 2005*. London: DoH.

Drummond, M.F. and Pang, F. (2001) Transferability of economic evaluations, in M.F. Drummond and A.J. McGuire (eds) *Economic Evaluation in Health Care: Merging Theory with Practice*. Oxford: Oxford University Press.

European Court of Justice (1998) Case C-158/96, *Kohll* v. *Union des Caisses de Maladie* and Case C-120/95, *Decker* v. *Caisse de maladie des employes prives*.

European Court of Justice (2001a) Case C-157/99, *Geraets-Smits* v. *Stichting Ziekenfonds VGZ* and *Peerbooms* vs. *Stichting CZ Groep Zorgverzekeringen*.

European Court of Justice (2001b) Case C-368/98 *Vanbraekel and others* v. *Alliance Nationale des Mutualites Chretinnes (ANMC)*.

Garrison, L. and Towse, A. (2003) The drug budget silo mentality in Europe: an overview, *Value in Health*, 6(suppl): S1–9.

Gatsios, K. and Seabright, P. (1989) Regulation in the European Community, *Oxford Review of Economic Policy*, 5(2): 37–60.

Healthcare Market News (2003) VII(XI): 206–8.

High Court of Justice Queen's Bench Division (2002) Case No CO/5690/2002, *Yvonne Watts* v. *Bedford Primary Care Trust and Secretary of State for Health*.

Hotelling, H. (1929) Stability in competition, *Economic Journal*, 39: 41–57.

Manca, A., Rice, N., Sculpher, M.J. and Briggs, A.H. (in press) Assessing generalisability by location in trial-based cost-effectiveness analysis: the use of multilevel models, *Health Economics*.

Maynard, A. (2002/3) Drug dealing and drug dependency, *Eurohealth*, 8(5): 8–10.

Nerb, G. (1988) *The Completion of the Internal Market: A Survey of European Industry's Perception of the Likely Effects*. Luxembourg: Office for Official Publications of the European Communities.

Rehnberg, C. (2002) A Swedish case study on the impact of the SEM on the pharmaceutical market, in R. Busse, M. Wismar and P.C. Berman (eds) *The European Union and Health Services*, pp. 131–58. Amsterdam: IOS Press.

Swann, D. (1995) *The Economics of the Common Market*. London: Penguin.

Szende, A., Mogyorosy, A., Muszbek, N., Nagy, J., Pallos, G. and Dozsa, C. (2002) Methodological guidelines for conducting economic evaluation of health care interventions in Hungary, *European Journal of Health Economics*, 3: 196–206.

Venables, A.J. (2003) Winners and losers from regional integration agreements, *The Economic Journal*, 113: 747–61.

HEALTH ECONOMICS AND HEALTH POLICY: A POSTSCRIPT

Peter C. Smith, Mark Sculpher and Laura Ginnelly

INTRODUCTION

This book has offered a necessarily selective but nevertheless wide-ranging survey of the potential contribution of economic analysis to emerging policy challenges in the domains of health and health care. The chapters cover a spectrum of policy problems and economic methodologies, ranging from the measurement of outcomes at the individual level to the whole-system concerns of finance and regulation. The book has identified some notable progress in the use of economic evidence for health policy. To take just some of the topics covered, one can point to remarkable advances in the methodology and policy impact of economic evaluation methods; routine adoption in many systems of health status measurement instruments; general acceptance of economic approaches towards capitation funding methods; and widespread experimentation with economic models of performance assessment. In short, economic analysis has made a major contribution to thinking about, and regulation of, health systems.

Celebration of such progress must, however, be tempered by the knowledge that there is so much more that can be done. This book has sought to explore some of the most fruitful ways forward. It carries some generic messages for both economists and policymakers, which we summarize briefly. We then mention some further challenges not covered by the book, and conclude by drawing together some general themes emerging from the preceding chapters.

FOR POLICYMAKERS

Our messages for policymakers are relatively straightforward. Inevitably we conclude that health policy is still often made in the absence of potentially useful economic evidence. The shortage of evidence is in part the fault of economists themselves, who have sometimes had a tin ear for the preoccupations of policymakers, failed to develop theory and analysis relevant to policy problems, and not made best use of increasingly extensive datasets. However, it is also the case that policymakers have failed to encourage researchers either directly (by financing appropriate research) or indirectly (by showing more engagement with potentially relevant research). Indeed, in the UK at least, the broader incentive regime for academic economists – with its emphasis on theory, methodological ingenuity and international focus – deliberately and strongly discourages the sort of empirical, interdisciplinary, carefully disseminated research that is likely to be useful for policy purposes.

Yet even where economic evidence is available in an accessible format, it is often ignored or used only selectively. For example, at the time of writing, English policymakers are introducing a major reform to the financing of hospitals, which will result in hospitals being funded almost entirely on the basis of centrally-determined case payments, using a form of diagnosis-related groups. While this reform may lead to some important gains, there is also ample international evidence to indicate that without some flexibility in the payment regime serious market instability and other adverse outcomes are likely to materialize. There are some clear indications as to how the proposed reform can be modified to accommodate these concerns. Yet, although these have been raised in very clear and practical terms by numerous commentators, policymakers appear reluctant to engage with the evidence in this particular respect.

More generally, certain oversimplified policy prescriptions from economic theory are sometimes seized upon by policymakers as a justification for policy initiatives, without regard for the detailed design issues on which success or failure will depend. An example is the promotion of markets and competition, among either purchasers or providers of health care, as a stimulus for performance improvement. When designed carefully, the introduction of competition into some parts of the health system can yield important benefits. Yet equally, as the US experience indicates, an indiscriminate reliance on markets can lead to gross inefficiency and inequity.

Researchers are often criticized for failing to communicate their evidence in a format that can be comprehended by policymakers. Certainly we need much better tools (and incentives) to improve our dissemination methods. But equally, there is an opportunity cost to dissemination, and researchers need to be confident that policymakers are listening and value their research. Many of the authors in this book have experimented with a variety of dissemination methods, yet have at times signally failed to secure any meaningful feedback – either positive or negative – from policymakers. Policy audiences need to become much better at telling researchers what formats of dissemination work best, and be more active in seeking out and engaging with research evidence.

Finally, policymakers can sometimes be myopic, failing to think beyond the boundaries of their own system. Yet there is often important evidence emerging from other health systems that can usefully be incorporated into domestic policy. Furthermore, health care is not immune to the rapid globalization of our economies (see Chapter 10), and policymakers must become increasingly alert to the implications of increased mobility of citizens, patients and workforces.

FOR ECONOMISTS

The book contains numerous challenges for health economists. Most directly, it suggests that there are important domains, such as the economic evaluation of health technologies, regulation and decentralization, where better theory is needed. To this end, there may be substantial benefits to looking across at other domains of economic enquiry, such as the mature literatures on industrial organization (see Chapter 5), income distribution (see Chapter 4), public finance (see Chapter 9) and evaluation of transport and environmental policies (see Chapter 1). More generally, health economics often seems to progress in isolation from developments in mainstream economic thought, and there are clear gains for health economists from drawing on relevant theoretical models as they emerge.

Conversely, there may be scope for some transfer of the ideas of health economics to other domains of economic enquiry. For example, the health status measurement instruments discussed in Chapter 2 offer a model for other areas of economic enquiry, many of which would benefit from more careful attention to measurement issues. Similarly, the relatively well-developed economic literature on equity in health might with benefit be applied to debates on equity in other public services, such as access to further and higher education. There are also important parallels between criminal justice systems and health systems. Criminal justice economics has not yet reached the state of maturity of its health counterpart, and in principle there appears to be great scope for applying some of the health economist's models to problems of policing, sentencing and rehabilitation.

From a situation only a few years ago of severe data limitations, the availability of quantitative information is being transformed in many aspects of modern health systems. This revolution in the scope, timeliness and quality of data offers hitherto unimagined opportunities for testing theories and designing policy instruments. Econometrics must therefore move to the centre of health economists' endeavours, and there is a need to ensure that the necessary skills and incentives to exploit the emerging opportunities are in place. Moreover, there is often a concern that empirical findings may not be transferable from one health system to another. Economists should prize replication of empirical studies in different health systems when the generalizability of results is questioned.

There are areas of enquiry where economics has hitherto had less influence than it perhaps should. To take just one example, many initiatives in public health are not subjected to the sort of rigorous economic evaluation that applies to more conventional health technologies. Certainly, the evaluation of population-based interventions raises many methodological challenges. They often yield benefits only over a long time horizon, and involve coordination with many agencies beyond the health system. However, if such initiatives are as crucial to health system performance as many believe, they need to be designed with a view to maximizing cost-effectiveness, using the same standards of evidence as we require of clinical interventions. There are clear opportunities for economists in this domain.

Other areas of research offering new opportunities have been specifically raised in the book. They include methods to prioritize the allocation of limited research resources. It continues to be the case that the bulk of research finance is allocated without explicit consideration of the limitations on research budgets. There is a need to be explicit about the objective of research and to use formal analytic methods to appraise the value of particular projects. Policymakers need to know where resources for health services research are best deployed, which methodologies secure the most cost-effective results, and the extent of economies of scope and scale in research. As discussed in Chapter 1, value of information methods represent a potentially valuable framework for the rational assessment of the efficiency of clinical research.

OTHER CHALLENGES

While we have sought to offer a broad survey of prospects, the book does not consider some important health policy issues. For example, at a micro level, there is increasing interest in the use of personal incentives for patients to use health services to best effect, and for the broader population to adopt healthy lifestyles. In the UK, the Wanless review of long-term trends in the NHS has highlighted the crucial role that a 'fully engaged' citizenry can play in securing a cost-effective health system. Economists clearly have a central role to play in the design and evaluation of appropriate incentive schemes.

The diffusion and take-up of new technologies varies considerably between developed countries, but our understanding of how and why those variations occur, and their link to system performance, is still rudimentary. There is need for engagement with other disciplines – such as organizational behaviour, psychology and sociology – to make much progress in this domain, but equally it is almost certainly the case that economists can make a major contribution.

As noted above, the explosion in availability of observational data offers the potential for enormous advances in the design and evaluation of policy initiatives. However, casual interpretation of observational data can be highly misleading. By modelling and interpreting system behaviour more carefully, econometric methodology, offers a crucial resource for moving beyond naïve analysis. Chapters 4 and 6 offer a glimpse of this potential in two specific domains (panel data and frontier estimation), but there is much more to be said on this topic.

Rapid changes in the way we live are giving rise to important new challenges. These are most obvious on the demand side, in the form (for example) of the potentially rapid spread of communicable diseases and the demands associated with an ageing population. On the supply side, new technologies such as genetic screening, nanotechnology and telemedicine may transform the way we need to think about the delivery of health care. These are all topics well suited to thoughtful economic analysis, again in conjunction with other disciplines.

Perhaps most importantly, we have chosen not to discuss the health policy problems confronted by developing countries. The problems of communicable diseases, human resources and financial constraints in low-income countries are some of the most serious global challenges confronted by mankind, and dwarf the preoccupations of the high-income countries discussed here. The discipline of economics clearly has an enormous potential contribution to make to health policy in low-income countries. However, we felt that the topic was so big and the challenges so distinct that we should leave it for another publication.

SOME GENERAL MESSAGES

In spite of the diversity of the topics covered, some common themes emerge from the book. We highlight just three. First, almost all the chapters reflect to a greater or lesser extent a concern with the equity of the health system, expressed in terms of financing, access and outcomes. Politicians have a natural concern with the pursuit of equity, as a perception of fairness is essential to securing widespread support for public finance of the health system. Yet policymakers are reluctant to articulate their equity concerns in a concrete fashion, or to state how far they feel equity should be pursued at the expense of efficiency. Furthermore, the equity concern underlying the debate in (say) the evaluation of technologies is not necessarily the same as that informing the fair financing debate. Economists have a major contribution to offer in helping policymakers make their intentions more explicit and relevant to operational decisions.

Second, many of the chapters suggest a need to develop economic thinking in conjunction with other disciplines, such as sociology, epidemiology, psychology, law, statistics, operational research, philosophy and medicine. Forty years of experience have demonstrated that policy prescriptions formulated purely in conventional economic terms are rarely adequate, and do not resonate with policymakers. But, equally, policies formulated without reference to economic principles – such as the enduring preoccupation with structural reorganization in the NHS – often have a high probability of failure. The clear message is that, however inconvenient, there must be a dialogue between disciplinary perspectives if many of the more wicked policy problems are to be addressed convincingly.

Third, we as editors have been struck by the interconnectedness of the issues being tackled in these chapters. While the concerns of economic evaluation, performance regulation, organizational structure and financing appear at first sight to require very different perspectives, they are all ultimately seeking to promote a more effective, efficient and equitable health system. Regrettably, health economists operating in one policy arena can often find themselves adopting a very narrow professional focus. For example, those of us evaluating health technologies rarely seek to integrate their work with those studying regulatory mechanisms. Yet we hope that this book has demonstrated that technology assessment should inform clinical guidelines and standards, which in turn should be reflected in the performance management and inspection regime. Finance systems should be designed to incentivize equitable and efficient implementation of chosen guidelines, and governance arrangements should be designed to offer the maximum local freedom and choice within the guideline regime. In short, our various areas of study are inextricably linked, and coherent system design should in principle be pursued in recognition of the links.

At present, most health systems have a long way to go if such coherence is to be achieved. In England, notwithstanding the efforts of NICE, many guidelines are promulgated without reference to economic evaluation. Where they are set, clinical standards can sometimes appear arbitrary, may fail to reflect patient heterogeneity, and are not always based on economic principles of cost-effectiveness. The performance management regime has tended to emphasize responsiveness, in particular waiting times, with little reference to clinical outcomes. Although capitation methods have reached an advanced stage of technical sophistication, there is little consideration of whether localities are being fairly financed to secure the increasing number of standards required of them. And, despite a stated commitment to devolve decision-making to local entities, central policymakers have found it difficult to break away from detailed operational prescription, and have failed to put in place adequate governance arrangements to ensure that local patients and citizens can make their preferences heard.

Such incoherence is in no way confined to England, and one could point to similar examples in almost all health systems. Indeed there is a sense in which it is only through the ambitious process of reform undertaken by English policymakers that the contradictions within the system have been exposed to the full glare of public scrutiny. What is needed now is a commitment to eliminate the more grotesque inconsistencies and inefficiencies, and we hope this book has indicated that economists can make a major contribution to that end.

CONCLUSIONS

There have in England alone been notable advances in bringing economic principles centre-stage in the creation and assessment of evidence for policy, the creation of NICE being the most dramatic example. Internationally, there are numerous parallel examples of the enduring and growing influence on policy of economic advisers in many health ministries, independent think-tanks and academia.

To some, the whole concept of 'health economics' might appear an oxymoron. What can the dismal science possibly contribute to health, that most fundamental of human goals? We hope that this book demonstrates that such a view is mistaken. While acknowledging that numerous disciplines must necessarily contribute to the development of good health policy, we believe that the economics perspective has a central role to play in improving the effectiveness, efficiency and equity of all health systems. At a parochial level, we hope that in 20 years' time our Centre continues to flourish. At a global level, we should hope to see that the fruitful collaboration between economics and policy has strengthened, and contributed to more cost-effective health systems everywhere.

INDEX

Page numbers for illustrations are shown in bold print

Related books from Open University Press
Purchase from www.openup.co.uk or order through your local bookseller

CULTURES FOR PERFORMANCE IN HEALTH CARE

Russell Mannion, Huw T.O. Davies and
Martin N. Marshall

- What is organizational culture?
- Do organizational cultures influence the performance of health care organizations?
- Are organizational cultures capable of being managed to beneficial effect?

Recent legislation in the United Kingdom has led to significant reforms within the health care system. Clinical quality, safety and performance have been the focus for improvement alongside systematic changes involving decision-making power being devolved to patients and frontline staff. However, as this book shows, improvements in performance are intrinsically linked to cultural changes within health care settings.

Using theories from a wide range of disciplines including economics, management and organization studies, policy studies and the health sciences, this book sets out definitions of cultures and performance, in particular the specific characteristics that help or hinder performance. Case studies of high and low performing hospital trusts and primary care trusts are used to explore the links between culture and performance. These studies provide examples of strategies to create beneficial, high-performance cultures that may be used by other managers. Moreover, implications for future policies and research are outlined.

Cultures for Performance in Health Care is essential reading for those with an interest in health care management and health policy including students, researchers, policy makers and health care professionals.

Contents
Series editor's introduction – List of figures and tables – List of boxes – About the authors – Foreword 1 by Aidan Halligan and Jay Bevington – Foreword 2 by Nigel Edwards – Acknowledgements – Introduction: policy background and overview – Making sense of organizational culture in health care – Does organizational culture influence health care performance? A review of existing evidence – Culture and performance in acute hospital trusts: integration and synthesis of case-study evidence – Culture and performance in English acute hospital trusts: condensed case study narratives – Findings from a quantitative analysis of all English NHS acute trusts – Findings from the primary care case studies – Summary, conclusions and implications for policy and research – Appendix 1 Research design and methods of data gathering and analysis – Appendix 2 Quantitative models and data definitions – References – Appendices.

256pp   0 335 21553 X (Paperback)   0 335 21554 8 (Hardback)